UNDER THE BANYAN TREE

UNDER THE BANYAN TREE

A Population Scientist's Odyssey

Sheldon J. Segal

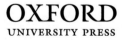

UNIVERSITY PRESS

2003

OXFORD
UNIVERSITY PRESS

Oxford New York
Auckland Bangkok Buenos Aires Cape Town Chennai
Dar es Salaam Delhi Hong Kong Istanbul Karachi Kolkata
Kuala Lumpur Madrid Melbourne Mexico City Mumbai
Nairobi São Paulo Shanghai Taipei Tokyo Toronto

Copyright © 2003 by Sheldon J. Segal

Published by Oxford University Press, Inc.
198 Madison Avenue, New York, New York 10016

www.oup.com

Oxford is a registered trademark of Oxford University Press

Library of Congress Cataloging-in-Publication Data
    Segal, Sheldon J. (Sheldon Jerome)
        Under the banyan tree : a population scientist's odyssey / Sheldon J. Segal.
        p. cm.
    Includes bibliographical references (p.).
    ISBN 0-19-515456-8
        1. Contraception. 2. Population research. 3. Population policy. 4. Social medicine.
    I. Title.
    RG136.S45 2002
    613.9'4—dc21   2002070393

9 8 7 6 5 4 3 2 1

Printed in the United States of America
on acid-free paper

Dedicated to The Population Council

Fifty Years of Excellence and Objectivity
     1952–2002

An institution that has fulfilled the expectations of its founder,
     John D. Rockefeller 3rd

Acknowledgments

I would like to thank many friends and colleagues who encouraged me to write this book for a general audience. Having written scientific articles for most of my career, it was not easy for me to write in the first person and include anecdotes about my own experiences to make a point. My wife, Harriet Segal, convinced me to do this and the idea was firmly endorsed by my friend and associate on the population odyssey, Elsimar Coutinho, and by my editor at Oxford University Press, Kirk Jensen. I hope my colleagues in the environmental and social sciences will not take it as hubris that a biomedical scientist delves into their disciplines to present the story that I think the public needs to learn about. The book is for people who want to understand the importance of population matters. Many people helped me when I had questions about issues in their fields. John Ross and John Bongaarts did some interesting and original calculations that I needed, and they helped me confirm many facts. Gavin Jones also checked my population statistics. I had similar assistance concerning ecology from Jerry Melillo of the Marine Biological Laboratory in Woods Hole. Thanks also to Martha Farnsworth Riche, former director of the U.S. Census Bureau, for her help. Anika Rahman, formerly of the Center for Reproductive Rights, provided me with valuable reference material. The center's founding president, Janet Benshoof, always inspires me to think about women's equality. Robert Herdt advised me on food production and agro-economics. Elof Johansson, Sab Koide, and Kalyan Sundaram responded without delay whenever I had questions for them. I share a sailboat with Luigi Mastroianni, which is indeed the true test of friendship. During hours on the *Sea Mast*, we discussed many of the issues I have written about, and he has always urged me to share my views with others. Thank you, Captain. I have a special feeling of gratitude to Gianna Celli and the staff of the Rockefeller Foundation's Conference and Study Center at Bellagio, Italy, on Lake Como. I include in my thanks the resident-scholars and other colleagues who shared the months Harriet and I spent at the Villa Serbelloni. Many ideas and clarifications of misconceptions came from our discussions. If you take this book home and read it, you'll quickly learn that much of it was written in Bellagio. My computer tells me I have mentioned it eight times in the twelve chapters. A final note of acknowledgment is owed to W. Parker Mauldin who was not around during the actual writing but who helped me understand demographic issues over the many years we worked together.

Contents

Introduction and Personal Note

The population of the world has now moved beyond 6 billion. It took all of human history to the mid-nineteenth century to reach the first billion. We are now adding almost 1 billion every 10 years. This comparison tells us that the world cannot sustain the present rate of growth for very long. Habitable land and resources are not unlimited. Sooner or later, birth rates will have to go down in regions where they remain high.

Don't let anybody tell you the increase in world population is over. Although it is true that fertility rates have been declining throughout much of the world, population expansion will continue well into this century. This is because growth is now due mainly to the momentum created by high birth rates of the recent past, which have resulted in record numbers of young people entering their reproductive years. Their sheer numbers will make up for the expected decline in fertility compared to their parents and grandparents.

Until recently the world could be divided between rich countries with low birth rates and poor countries with high birth rates. This is no longer the case. Many of the world's less developed countries in which annual income is well below the poverty level by any standard now have lower fertility rates.

Why did this drop in fertility take place? In the mid 1960s, less than 10% of couples in developing countries used some form of contraception. By 2000, use had risen to nearly 60%. Because a country's fertility rate is strongly correlated with contraceptive use, birth rates have dropped in places with traditionally high fertility. Women in India during the 1960s, for example, had an average of more than six children in their lifetime. This statistic is called the total fertility rate. Now, in India, the average number of children per woman is below four and falling. The United Nations predicts that it will drop down to about two by 2020. Reduction of the total fertility rate in China, the other population giant, has been even more rapid, urged along by a government policy that some Western critics consider excessively coercive.

When China announced its "one child per couple" policy in 1979, the government's Minister of Science and Technology, Fang Yi, explained to me that each year a staggering total of 20 million people were being added to a labor force already underemployed and shifting into cities as farming declined as a proportion of the country's total productivity. This, he told me, could not continue if stability was to be maintained in the country. Expecting foreign criticism, he asked me to convey the message that the new policy is a sacrifice that the present generation of Chinese must make for future generations. More than 20 years have passed since I had that conversation with Fang Yi, and China's total fertility rate has now fallen below replacement level. This means that the average Chinese couple limits childbearing to less than two children, even when the calculation includes minorities or rural families without a son, for whom the one child policy has never been strictly enforced.

China's population story is part of a remarkable change in human behavior during the last half of the twentieth century, facilitated by government-supported and government-implemented national family planning programs. Demographers and economists debate over the relative roles of societal factors on the one hand and the family planning movement on the other in the magnitude and timing of fertility declines, but the availability of family planning methods was essential regardless of the motivation that led to using them.

It was my privilege to play a role in this movement, first as the director of the biomedical efforts of the Population Council, a nonprofit research organization with laboratories located at New York's Rockefeller University, then as an officer of the Rockefeller Foundation. As a biomedical scientist representing these respected institutions over the past 45 years, my work has taken me to 68 countries on all continents, and I've had the opportunity to advise world leaders on matters pertaining to population, women's health, and, of course, family planning. In China, for example, as its forceful program got underway, I urged government leaders to accept the principle that $Q + V = S$, where Q = quality of family planning services, V = voluntarism, and S = success. Everywhere I traveled in rural China, the word seemed to precede me and colorful signs in English and Chinese would greet me announcing: Quality Plus Voluntarism Equals Success! When a symposium was held in Beijing so that health ministry officials from all the provinces of China could learn about the successful pilot projects we had sponsored in Hebei and Shangdong provinces, the slogan was festooned on the banner that was draped atop the speaker's stage.

One of my early assignments for the Population Council was in India to help start a Department of Reproductive Physiology in a new medical school and advise the government on contraceptive methods it could introduce in its emerging family planning program. For my wife and me, living in India changed our lives in ways we could not have imagined. We learned about the economically deprived world and the needs of its people. The experience changed my outlook toward my own work. Instead of focusing exclusively on basic science and publishing scientific journal articles, I have devoted my career to using science to develop practical advances for women's health. Advancing contraceptive technology is part of that; so is safe motherhood; and so is protection against sexually transmitted diseases including HIV/AIDS.

The era of national family planning began in India under Prime Minister Nehru shortly after the end of British rule. Through all subsequent administrations, family planning has been retained as an official government policy. It has been a political campaign issue occasionally, but only to criticize an incumbent government for ineffectiveness, never to suggest that the program should be abandoned.

Following the Indian lead, the movement was taken up by the eastern Asian countries of the Pacific rim, swept through South Asia, across the fertile crescent to North Africa, and to the countries of Latin America and the Caribbean. During the closing decades of the twentieth century, more than 90% of people in the less developed regions of the world lived in countries where government responsibility to provide their citizens with birth control services was accepted policy. The countries of sub-Saharan Africa tended to lag behind both in acceptance of family planning and in performance once programs were started.

When the family planning movement began, the technology of contraception was extremely limited. Political daring was needed to announce and undertake a program based on fertility beads and other primitive methods. You've never heard of fertility beads? They were an American invention by an "expert" who apparently had never been to India. The idea was to give women an attractive necklace with green and red beads. Each day of the month she was to move one bead, and when she came to the red beads, it was the signal that she could get pregnant. It was the calendar method in beads for illiterate village women. There were a few problems. Distributed as a gift, many women thought the necklace was too beautiful a possession to be worn every day so they would hide it away. When worn by a young mother, her nursing baby would move beads around playing with them. If she hung them in a tree out of her infant's reach, baby monkeys would play with them. And, of course, it was based on the naive assumption that women in male-dominated India controlled their own reproductive freedom. It's easy to see why Raj Kumari Amrit Kar, independent India's first Health Minister, a princess and disciple of Mahatma Gandhi, responded to the advice of Dr. Leona Baumgartner, New York City's Health Commissioner on a mission to India, by saying, "Yes, we know we need to provide family planning services to our people. Now tell me what we should offer them!"

The chances of success changed and the movement toward adopting family planning as a governmental activity hastened as science achieved the contraceptive advances of the past 40 years, beginning with the first oral contraceptive, "the pill," and the modern IUD (intrauterine device).

Contraceptive development is but one of the scientific inputs that have had a profound influence on the development and implementation of population policies. Other biomedical specialties as well as the social sciences have played key roles in the evolution of population policies from apathy to active government participation in educational and service programs. Water sanitation and other public health measures drastically reduced infant and child mortality. Surveys of knowledge, attitudes, and practice (KAP studies) helped many countries formulate policy and design family planning programs. Economists factored in demographic issues in formulating sustainable development policies.

Good science is sometimes displaced by political expediency in guiding public policy. I have written this book with the hope that it will enhance public interest and enlighten population dialogue. The present federal administration in Washington, D.C., holds views on population-related issues that are sharply different from those of the previous administration, and discussions of these differences have faded from public attention. Surprisingly, although Japan had volunteered to serve as host nation, preparation for a United Nations (U.N.) population conference in 2004 has been abandoned.

The United Nations has sponsored a series of population conferences. The first was held in Bucharest in 1974. These decennial events serve as important benchmarks that help trace the evolution of population policy and politics. The last U.N. population conference, officially called the International Conference on Population and Development (ICPD), was held in Cairo in 1994. Its intent was to address population concerns in terms of their interrelationships with economic growth, sustainable development, poverty alleviation, gender equality, and reproductive health.

Out of Cairo came a consensus report embracing a comprehensive approach to population and development. The ICPD Program of Action emphasized that sustainable development must take into account health issues including access to family planning services and human rights including reproductive rights. Inclusion of concern for reproductive rights recognized the rights of all women to decide freely on the number, spacing, and timing of their children and emphasized that they had the right to the means to do so free of discrimination, coercion, and violence. No one should overlook the importance of the clear articulation of this principle by the international community. The "Cairo agenda," as the conference's recommendations have come to be known, focuses unambiguously on the issues of women's human rights including reproductive rights, health, and empowerment.

With little to say about demographic issues, the Cairo conference on population emphasized access to reproductive health services and enhancing women's education, status, and opportunities. Empower women to exercise personal autonomy concerning their sexual and reproductive health, the message of Cairo said, and they'll take care of population as an integral part of both individual and broader development goals.

I welcomed the affirmation that development strategy and population considerations should address women's needs and emphasize the necessity to rectify intolerable injustices. The Cairo agenda gave primacy to the individual well-being rationale for population policies and family planning, the principle that has guided me throughout my career. It had another beneficial outcome by enhancing the status of the women's empowerment movement so that it could have a greater role in influencing policies in many countries, including our own.

The momentum toward gender equality was reinforced the following year by the World Conference on Women in Beijing and the Social Summit in Copenhagen. What happened at Cairo was important and indelible. Post-conference discussions continued to emphasize as the centerpiece of population policy improving the education, health, and status of women, facing up to gender inequality including society's ugly secret—unpunished violence toward women. These issues became "the new paradigm."

Moreover, the U.N. Population Fund (UNFPA), the organizing sponsor, came away from the Cairo conference heralding it as a landmark consensus on a comprehensive approach to population and development. UNFPA plays the leading role in the U.N. system in promoting population programs. Its purpose is to respond to needs in population and family planning and to help countries develop strategies to deal with them. This is why UNFPA's unqualified endorsement of the new paradigm—putting the spotlight on women's health, empowerment, and equality—had great significance. Five years after Cairo, in 1999 and 2000, review meetings around the world and at a special session of the U.N. General Assembly once again confirmed the essential elements of the Cairo agenda. It was a concept whose time has come to stay.

But there are other implications of the Cairo agenda, intended or unintended, that deserve attention. Not long before the Cairo meeting, UNFPA had issued comprehensive reports directed to the themes that economic advances in developing countries and environmental problems are often linked to population growth. One preconference UNFPA report argued that rapid population growth impedes the development process and exacerbates deficiencies in health, education, and malnutrition. Another addressed the fact that rapid population growth contributes to global environmental problems such as deforestation and air or water pollution.

These U.N. reports constitute just a small sampling of the scientific and academic literature on consequences of population growth. The report out of the Cairo meeting gave scant attention to these matters. Consequently, instead of amplifying discussions of population matters, Cairo had a dampening effect on the level of dialogue. Important population issues faded from the radar screen of public concern.

Moreover, after the Cairo conference, a new term with a pejorative connotation entered the lexicon of influential advocates of the new paradigm. The catchword to describe the consequences of rapid population growth was the "demographic imperative." It became a shibboleth to describe the use of demographic arguments as the basis for establishing population policy. If, for example, a country is concerned about low fertility and offers bonuses to *encourage* child-bearing, this would be policy driven by a demographic imperative. My example, of course, is the opposite of the actual target of post-Cairo critics—policymaking with a demographic objective to *lower* fertility. The implication was that concern about world population numbers or the consequences of rapid population growth was not only out of date, but an indication that "you just don't get it."

Signs of the schism were evident even earlier than the Cairo conference. As Vice President Al Gore prepared to lead the American delegation to the Rio de Janeiro Conference on Environment and Development in 1992, word got out that the U.S. position paper would include a comment on the relationship between population and environment. A meeting of feminist leaders was hastily organized at the Ford Foundation's headquarters in New York. It seemed logical that the linkage between population growth and environmental issues should be discussed at Rio. But there was adamant opposition. I recall one particularly angry speaker who declared that, "we will not allow them to claim in Rio that environmental degradation begins in the uterus of women!" This was a strange interpretation of Gore's position and created an even stranger coalition: American feminists and the Vatican, which also wanted to keep population off the Rio agenda. One group wanted to put an end to considering women as targets in the implementation of population and environment policies, the other group wanted to promote its religious teachings under the banner of addressing human needs.

What struck me both during the pre-Rio debates and after Cairo was the single-issue mentality of those whom I admired for their devotion to improving the status, health, and position of women throughout the world. For many of the leaders in the struggle for gender equality, the only rationale for population policy became the new paradigm of Cairo. A broader agenda, based on scientific analysis of the impact of population growth on other human affairs (the demographic imperative) was disregarded and even scorned.

I was amazed to observe how the rise of the new paradigm diluted concern about issues that the UNFPA had described shortly before the Cairo meeting. Attention to decades of policy analysis and data collection by economists, demographers, geographers, and other scientific experts seemed to be diminished.

The primary importance of improving the welfare of the individual has been a cornerstone of the population movement. John D. Rockefeller 3rd, the Population Council's founder, used a phrase in many of his speeches that expressed his deeply held conviction: "Our concern is for the quality of human life, not the quantity of human life." Personally, this is the rationale that attracted me to the population field.

From time to time I have been asked, "If you have one dollar to spend on family planning, what would you do?" My answer is simple, "Put it into educating young girls." Experience in developing countries has taught me that little girls frequently do not attend school with their brothers. They are not in the classroom, but kept home for domestic tasks like gathering wood, carrying water, or collecting cow dung to be dried and used for fuel. But my point of view was not necessarily shared by other influential figures in the family planning movement, who preferred to concentrate resources on contraceptive saturation programs. They seemed to have a dogged concern for numbers rather than for people and their needs—numbers of contraceptives distributed, numbers of "acceptors," numeric targets met. Women were seen as objects through which to implement population programs and policies. Evidently this was the extremist viewpoint that polarized positions and created the sharp delineation of purpose in the Cairo agenda.

When Dr. Halfdan Mahler was director-general of the World Health Organization in the 1980s, he described the risk of pregnancy-associated death in poor countries compared to rich countries as the most obscene of all health statistics differences. A caring person cannot disagree. An infant girl born in the United States or Canada, for example, has 1 chance in 8000 of dying of a pregnancy-related cause during her lifetime. In some African countries the lifetime risk is 1 in 20.

Driven by this outrageous inequality, many of us in the population community formed an effective coalition with women's health advocates to promote safe motherhood. In my role as director of the Rockefeller Foundation's Population Sciences program, I had guided the foundation in a balanced approach toward women's health and other population matters including subjects such as contraceptive development and demographic research and training. It was not uncharacteristic, therefore, that the Rockefeller Foundation was the first nongovernmental donor to pledge funds for the World Health Organization to start a formal program to promote safe motherhood and to study practical ways to reduce maternal mortality in high-risk situations. Other projects we supported included entrepreneurial training and micro-loans for village women.

Before the Cairo conference, I believed that such collaborations had established a healthy partnership linking thoughtful advocacy for women's equality and health with the scientific analysis of the causes and consequences of population growth. It surprised me that Cairo did not reinforce the merits of this partnership. Major philanthropic foundations with a history of leadership in the population field and in women's health shifted focus and began to decline applications for support of projects concerned with the demographic imperative because this subject was no longer within their program guidelines.

Foundations with longstanding programs in population, Ford, MacArthur, and Rockefeller, joined this trend. The Ford Foundation had already given up its population program by 1994. The venerable Rockefeller Foundation, after a year of study and consultations, dropped population as a program theme and adopted for its population-related activities in 2000 the title "Implementing the Cairo Agenda."

I often wonder if trustees who are concerned about world population growth and believe the foundations they govern have a population program realize the extent to which the new paradigm has replaced initiatives concerned with other global, national, and local challenges of population growth. I corresponded about this with a good friend in academia. His reaction was that interest in these demographic concerns had waned or been replaced by more immediate human needs, and raising them would only be boring for policy makers and political leaders in developing countries. I was not convinced because I had just returned from India where the newspapers were full of stories about the intensifying problem of air pollution linked with the growth of cities like Mumbai (formerly Bombay) and Calcutta.

I can more easily understand the rationale that the new paradigm, enhancing women's empowerment, is not a change in the ultimate objectives of population policies but in the means to achieve them. The premise is that enabling women to achieve personal autonomy over their own reproductive aims is an intrinsic right and will reduce fertility rates as well as improve the quality of life for women, their families, and communities. Moreover, there is substantial evidence to support this conclusion. In countries where studies have been done, a higher level of mother's education correlates well with lower fertility. Average age of marriage increases with increasing level of education. Surveys find that even at prevailing educational levels for women, desired family size runs below actual fertility rates in many developing countries. This reflects the unmet need for contraception.

I have no doubt that efforts to increase women's self-determination will improve the health and well-being of women and their children and can slow the pace of population growth. Even if the evidence weren't compelling, working to eliminate inequities facing women throughout the world deserves high priority for its own sake. In short, promoting a just world for women can produce a better world.

The population field's new paradigm after the Cairo conference of 1994 was the result of a long evolutionary process with considerable scientific input. The concept had already left its imprint on the recommendations of previous U.N. conferences of the early 1990s on education, environment, health, and children. The movement toward gender equality and the empowerment of women had its roots in modern feminism, women's studies, and other social science research. The public health profession also played an important role in defining principles of links between health and human rights and appropriate and effective programs for women.

Critics who chose to define family planning as simply handing out contraceptive supplies did not appreciate the extent to which a greater understanding of what women wanted and needed had evolved in the earliest days of family planning programs. The first family-planning field worker I ever visited was Swedish gynecologist Arne Kinch, who was working in a health center outside of Colombo, Ceylon (now Sri

Lanka) supported by the Swedish International Development Agency. We spent the hours talking about cervical cancer, Pap smears, infertility, and the day-to-day problems he faced with the women he was trying to help. Later, when I moved to nearby India, we arranged an air shipment service using the Ford Foundation's small Cessna (these were the pre-FedEx days) so that he could send Pap smears to New Delhi where we had the diagnostic lab that he didn't have in Colombo.

The past-director of UNFPA, Dr. Nafis Sadik, a Pakistani physician, made her mark on the international scene by her visionary policy of comprehensive advancement of woman's health as the keystone of her country's family planning program early in its history.

Even at the first U.N. Population Conference in Bucharest in 1974, the seeds of family planning as a component of women's health were evident. Although overshadowed by political positioning and tensions between donor and recipient countries, the U.N. report included the recommendation of integrating family planning services into maternal health programs. At Bucharest, the American delegation, representing the Nixon/Ford administration, emphasized the drag on development efforts caused by a rapid rate of population growth and encouraged developing countries to set demographic targets and give greater priority to family planning. But there was suspicion about the motives behind the generous foreign aid offered by the United States and other rich countries.

This was evident in discussions I had with young Asian and African doctors who served in primary health centers in small villages. They resented the fact that once family planning assistance started, their dispensaries might always be well stocked with contraceptives, but they could never be sure about supplies of bandages, antibiotics, or other medicines. (This problem persists today. A Ugandan doctor told me recently that in rural western Uganda, to replenish supplies a health clinic worker must get on a bicycle and travel to a distant supply center and then make the long walk back pushing the cycle with the supply box strapped to the seat—provided the needed medicines were available. The same worker watches enviously as each month a gleaming four-wheel-drive vehicle, donated by UNFPA, drives up to deliver the monthly supply of contraceptives. When I repeated this to a senior Ghanaian physician, he confirmed that the same situation still prevails in his country.)

Understandably, the concerns of the young doctors were reflected in the official positions taken by their country delegations at Bucharest back in 1974. The representative of India, Health Minister Karan Singh, startled the United States delegates by countering their hard-sell for birth control with the phrase that captured the attention of the international press corps and has lived on as the legacy of the Bucharest conference: "Development is the best contraceptive." (Frustrated by the continuing poverty in his country 30 years later, now-retired Karan Singh has recently written, "Contraception is the best development.")

That meeting of nations to discuss population in 1974 resulted in a first-ever World Population Plan of Action. This led to the 1984 Mexico City Declaration on Population and Development, sensitive to both women's health needs and the necessity for equality in the role and status of women. It stated, "population and development policies should strive to hasten the complete equality of women in social, economic and political life," and emphasized that special attention should be given to maternal and child health services.

The difference between these earlier pronouncements and the Cairo agenda was commitment and emphasis. In Bucharest, more press attention was given to the speech-making at the concurrent forum of nongovernmental agencies than to the press releases from the governmental conference.

It was in Bucharest that Population Council founder and trustee John Rockefeller questioned the effectiveness in economic development of "family planning alone." I was not present to hear his speech, but I later learned that the council's president, Bernard Berelson, and others were surprised and even dismayed, not because they disagreed but because they couldn't understand where he got the idea that family planning stood alone as a strategy to reduce poverty. It could not have been from his familiarity with the council's diversified program on population, health, and development in which family planning was included, but not as a component that stood alone. Berelson, for example, had just launched the now renowned international journal, *Population and Development Review* (*PDR*), which covers economic themes and analyses far afield from the idea that family planning alone would be a solution to economic development. The dimensions of population policy and the two-way relationships between population and socioeconomic development had been recognized for a long time. With his characteristic wry humor, distinguished economist and *PDR* editor Paul Demeny once described family planning programs under circumstances unprepared for such services as equivalent to "opening a Polish restaurant in an Italian neighborhood."

Nevertheless, Rockefeller's council colleagues enthusiastically applauded his call for greater attention to the role of women in development efforts, a subject on which he proved to be a visionary. (Recently, pioneer feminist Betty Friedan told me that she was invited to meet with Rockefeller before Bucharest and discussed with him her view that women did not need contraceptives as much as they needed education and better health care. I had not known of that meeting before. It probably was an important element in shaping John Rockefeller's evaluation and the famous phrase of his Bucharest speech.)

Ten years later, in August 1984, at the next U.N. Conference on Population at Mexico City, many countries came with a political agenda not directly related to the subject of the conference. Queen Noor of Jordan, for example, used the podium as her country's delegate to speak on behalf of Palestinians living in refugee camps. The Vatican delegation lobbied hard against abortion, then a political issue before the Mexican legislature. With the Mexico City event coming just before the 1984 elections, the U.S. delegation appointed by President Ronald Reagan used the conference to make its own domestic political points.

In the decade from Bucharest to Mexico City, there was a complete role reversal between the United States and developing countries. In Mexico City, the U.S. delegation, following the Reagan administration's policy, declared that population was a neutral factor with respect to economic development. This reversed the position held by every president since Dwight Eisenhower. The new U.S. position elicited opposition from developing country delegates who came to Mexico City prepared to adopt in the plan of action a strong position in support of family planning in the context of population and development. A vote on the issue found that 1 country out of the 148 member nations agreed with the United States: North Yemen. The daily newspaper published for the conference delegates ran a cartoon the following day showing Uncle Sam as a fat-cat capitalist handing out cigars to poor people and encouraging them to have more babies. It was biting humor that seemed to amuse everyone except the American delegation.

The head of the delegation was former Conservative Party Senator James Buckley of New York, and his deputy was Allan Keyes, the ardent abortion opponent who later became a familiar and articulate candidate for president in Republican Party primaries and now a television personality. The highlight of Buckley's speech, and the item stressed in the delegation's press release, was a new antiabortion component to U.S. foreign assistance. This was the famous Mexico City policy or global gag rule that would deprive U.S. government support to any agency, American or foreign, that used its own funds to support abortion services, counseling, or referral, even though providing these services might be perfectly legal in the country concerned and no U.S. money was involved. The global gag rule prevailed through the Reagan and Bush years, was dropped five days after President Bill Clinton was sworn in, and reestablished three days after President George W. Bush took office.

As the delegates and guests were leaving the meeting room immediately after the Buckley speech, a U.S. television anchorman interviewed Faye Wattleton, president of Planned Parenthood Federation of America, who expressed her dismay. A leader in the antiabortion movement who happened to be a physician elbowed his way forward. On camera, he was asked if he was satisfied with the U.S. position paper. His answer was, "It was a good first step." "What is the next step?" was the reporter's follow-up question. "Now the United States has to stop all those abortions caused by contraceptives, like the pill and the IUD," he replied. When I was asked to comment, I did not hesitate to say that his statement astonished me, not only because of its lack of scientific credibility, but because it revealed the true extent of his opposition to women's reproductive rights. It did not stop at abortion. It included contraception as well. My public position earned me a vulgar demonstration by pro-lifers at the banquet given by the Secretary General of the United Nations in honor of the U.N. Population Award Laureates the following evening.

In the debate on the Mexico City Plan of Action, the Swedish delegation urged that the problem of women dying because of illegal and unsafe abortions must be addressed, and some statement should be included acknowledging the problem. The Swedish recommendation neither endorsed nor recommended legalization of abortion. It was simply a plea that the conference recognize that unsafe abortion is a serious cause of death and injury to women throughout the world. But the United States opposed any mention of abortion in the final document, even in this context of concern for the health of women. The American delegation turned a deaf ear to the Swedish appeal for concern about the millions of women each year who end unwanted pregnancies, often in circumstances that are unsafe, costing many of them their lives and leaving their young children motherless. Once again, the U.S. position garnered just one ally. This time it was the Vatican. Ultimately, compromise terminology was included in the conference's final report which begrudgingly acknowledged that women who have had recourse to abortion should receive counseling and be treated humanely.

I was honored to receive the U.N. Population Award at Mexico City as a co-recipient with the distinguished Panamanian demographer Carmen Miro. The previous awards had gone to political leaders, Indira Gandhi, prime minister of India, and Qian Xinzhong, the president of China. The selection of a social scientist and a biomedical scientist for this honor was a first, and it earned us the opportunity to address the conference. My remarks reflected none of the opinions expressed by the official U.S. position paper or in Buckley's speech. I emphasized reproductive freedom to give couples greater control over their lives and over the hopes and aspirations for their children. I was by no means alone in these contrary views. The sentiments I expressed reflected the attitude of many of my colleagues in the population field, even if they were not shared by my country's delegation. Moreover, the position papers of many delegations emphasized the relationship between rapid population growth and economic development, the individual well-being objective of population policies, and included statements about integrating family planning services into more comprehensive women's health programs. This was welcome news to me. While living in India, I helped the Ministry of Health design model family planning clinics that promoted pre- and postnatal visits, nutrition programs for low-weight infants, as well as women's health services, including infertility consultations, diagnosis and treatment of reproductive tract infections, and cancer screening. My naiveté about Health Ministry budgets did not dampen my enthusiasm for the diversity of what should be included in family planning services.

One of the unforgettable memories of my career was holding an infertility clinic in rural India with Anna Southam, a gynecologist from the medical school faculty of Columbia University. In New Delhi, professors and health ministry officials tried to talk us out of it, saying we would be wasting our time; the villagers would not bring so personal a problem as infertility to strangers, particularly foreigners. We went anyway. The village couples came, husband and wife together, from great distances when they learned that foreign experts had come to the district family health clinic to try to help them.

One successful pregnancy came out of those consultations, thanks to Dr. Southam's surgical intervention the following day under amazingly primitive circumstances with an ether cone for anesthesia and a gooseneck lamp for illuminating the surgical field. Only a few of the men had subfertile sperm counts, the part of the clinic that was my responsibility. I was surprised because I expected to find the infertility causes to be about 50:50 between the husbands and wives. No one declined to provide a semen sample, contrary to the Delhi predictions. The main cause for infertility was something long gone from the clinical scene in the United States: tuberculosis of the endometrium. There were occasional light moments during a long and hard day. One couple, both well-educated, were teachers who worked in different parts of India and only got together when they returned to their village for "a fortnight vacation." Anna explained through our interpreter, Dr. Sabita Sujan, that if they wanted to make a baby, they would have to do better than that!

But even in those early years of family planning programs, I was just one among many who understood the need to emphasize all aspects of women's health as a part of family planning. India's director of family planning, Dr. B. L. Raina, a retired army colonel, had little patience for the health clinic bureaucrats who assigned consultation rooms separately labeled "Family Planning" and "Maternal Health." When we went on tour together and encountered clinics with this situation, his military background would become evident, and there would be no backtalk as he ordered the necessary changes in order to integrate the two. My mentor on public health in India, Dr. Moye Freymann, and I were frequently at odds with officers of bilateral assistance agencies, especially our own U.S. Agency for International Development, who interpreted family planning assistance to mean providing contraceptive supplies.

This is not to say that distribution of contraceptives was not a part of family planning from the onset. At another Indian village, meeting with the local youth club, Anna Southam and I asked if they had any questions after our description of methods of birth control. The response was, "You foreign people always come and tell us about these things. When are you going to bring some?"

The road from Bucharest through Mexico City to Cairo followed a constant course to bring women's issues into the context of population policy. It finally came into clear focus and prominence in Cairo. But along the way, conference deliberations did not disregard the consequences of demographic issues or criticize attention to these matters. My own target for criticism of population policies and family planning measures through the years has been the imposing of the will of donor countries on the programs of recipient countries and the use of coercive measures by governments believing that the urgency of their country's population problem justified any means to stop women from having babies.

Throughout my association with the Population Council and the Rockefeller Foundation, our position was absolute and unalterable opposition to the use of coercion in family planning programs. We disagreed with the use of sterilization camps, gifts of transistor radios, or cash bonuses for "finders" who brought people to vasectomy clinics. I let this be known in my frequent trips to developing countries, so there was never any question of our either initiating or participating in family planning efforts that involved coercion.

The subject of incentive schemes to increase acceptance of contraceptives was on the agenda of a meeting I attended before the Bucharest Conference of 1974. Sponsored by the Ford Foundation and held at the Villa d'Este on Italy's Lake Como, the purpose of the meeting was to discuss foreign assistance to national family planning programs. We agreed that aid should not be given for coercive measures and were attempting to define how to draw the line between coercion and the application of persuasive marketing techniques. Was it coercion to reimburse deeply impoverished people for the hypothetical cost of travel to a clinic or for time lost from nonexistent jobs? The distinctions between persuasion, incentive, and coercion seemed impossible to agree on. I argued that even the perception of coercion was unacceptable. To emphasize my point, I paraphrased my mentor, the Population Council's retired president and esteemed Princeton demographer Frank Notestein, that coercion or the perception of coercion will bring down a government before it brings down the birth rate! How prophetic this proved to be when Prime Minister Indira Gandhi failed to be returned to office by the voters of India when she confidently called a special election in March 1977. Analysts believe that the imposition of coercive family planning measures under the influence and advice of her younger son, Sanjay, contributed heavily to Mrs. Gandhi's defeat.

Foreign aid for family planning is not high on the priority list of

American voters. Nevertheless, I thought it would be important in 1984 to learn how well the positions that were going to be announced by Buckley and the U.S. delegation at the Mexico City Conference matched with those of the American people. We commissioned a Gallup poll to answer this question, and I presented the results at a press conference the day before the opening of the U.N. conference. The results showed that the Reagan policy did not represent the views of the people of the United States. A substantial majority of the Americans polled disagreed with his stance against abortion rights, opposed the imposition of restrictions on U.S. assistance to family planning programs, and did not support the view that population is a nonissue for the economic development of poor countries. In fact, not a single point in the United States position paper won public support. One would have liked to believe that the delegation sent to an international conference represented the national viewpoint. In our poll we found that most of the American people favored the provision of contraceptive supplies as part of the government's foreign assistance program and a majority opposed the so-called global gag rule.

In 1998 a survey done by Rand Corporation using almost identical questions showed that the attitudes of Americans have not changed on these issues. More than 70% believe that too much population growth in developing countries is holding back their economic development. Eighty percent favor U.S. foreign assistance for voluntary family planning programs in developing countries. More than half of Americans polled in 1998 disapprove of the U.S. withholding funds for family planning services to health organizations if these organizations also provide abortion services with other, non-U.S. funding. This question did not include the fact that funds could be withheld if counseling and referrals without actual abortion procedures were provided. Nor did it clarify that providing abortion services with U.S. funds is already prohibited under the Helms Amendment that is included each year in the U.S. AID appropriations bill. Perhaps the margin of disapproval would have increased with this information.

Ten years after the Mexico City meeting, a significant difference was the important role given to nongovernmental organizations and individuals in formulating the U.S. position and in participation at the Cairo conference. The Clinton administration's chief delegate, former senator and cabinet member Tim Wirth, took with him to Cairo a team that represented diverse views on population, women's health, and economic development. It was in the true spirit of representative government, a delegation that represented the American people. Wirth's team played a major role in formulating the Cairo agenda, and the American position had little trouble in gaining nearly unanimous support among the 185 participating nations.

The George W. Bush administration's positions on population-related matters appear to be a reprise of the Reagan/Bush Mexico City policy of 1984. The U.S. delegation did not acknowledge the relevance of population matters at the September 2002 Earth Summit in Johannesburg. In fact, the president chose not to attend. There will also be U.N. conferences on children, on food and hunger, on women, and on climate change. We can expect similar avoidance of population issues as the U.S. participates in these U.N. conferences. I hope this book will help to sustain the population dialogue so that the American public can better understand some of the scientific issues involved. I have enjoyed my adventures in population research and share them with you to enhance this understanding.

When I began my personal odyssey as a population scientist, I was forewarned by friends and by Paul Ehrlich's book, *The Population Bomb*, to steel myself for the misery and poverty I would encounter on my first trip to India. Instead, there is an image of India that has stayed with me as a lasting memory: the children of an Indian village sitting in the shade of a large banyan tree, holding their slates on their laps, looking up eagerly as they listened to their teacher in that schoolroom provided by nature. I didn't realize it at the time, but those pupils, boys and girls, held the key that will eventually release their country from poverty and subsistence living. The educational transition, symbolized by the banyan tree, from illiteracy to mass schooling, proves to be the prior condition to the demographic transition from high to low fertility and the economic transition to rising income and affluence. In the process, girls cannot be left behind.

Emphasizing the important of education, however, does not imply a disregard for the demographic imperative—a greater understanding of the consequences of population growth. I hope this book contributes constructively to the discussions on how population issues affect the human condition and the planet that we must preserve for generations that will follow us. There is room under the banyan tree for all who share this common goal.

UNDER THE BANYAN TREE

1

The Changing World Population

We see the world in terms of the human experience. It is always changing. Neither the quality nor the quantity of human life is a constant.

In the fourteenth century, when the world had about 450 million inhabitants, a quarter of the people of Europe were wiped out by the bubonic plague. The future must have seemed bleak to survivors. Two hundred years later, Elizabethan literature flourished, European explorers had discovered the New World, and population had inched up to 550 million. Until the advent of disease prevention, high death rates kept the population growth rate in check. Over the centuries, smallpox alone took hundreds of millions of lives, but by the eighteenth century, with the emergence of science during the Enlightment, medical advances such as Jenner's vaccine and the germ theory of disease led to lower death rates and faster growth of population numbers.

The milestone of 1 billion in world population was reached around 1800. The history of population growth during the 1800s and 1900s was an accelerating pace of increase. When the calendar closed on the twentieth century, the earth had 6 billion inhabitants, 2–3 billion living in poverty on $1 or $2 a day, many barely surviving on what they can eke out from the earth around them. In some regions that number is growing. There is a great divide between the rich and the poor and that too is growing. The total consumption expenditures of the world's population living in industrialized countries is over 17 trillion U.S. dollars while developing countries, with more than 80% of the world's people, record consumption expenditures of about 5 trillion dollars. In rich countries, more than 99% of children reach their fifth birthday; in poor countries more than 20% do not. Rich countries, with about 20% of world population, consume nearly 60% of the world's total energy resources; the poorest 20% of people in poor countries use less than 4%.

With fertility rates in many countries still far above replacement levels, and large numbers of young people entering their reproductive years, rapid increase in population is continuing. At present, we are adding nearly a billion every decade, almost entirely in the world's poorest regions. Each minute more than 100 people are added—nearly 150,000 every day. As I write these pages in Bellagio, Italy, looking over picturesque Lake Como, we receive news of the terrible, tragic loss of life in the Indian earthquake on the country's Republic Day, 2001. We read press reports that the fatality toll may reach 100,000. Aside from the human tragedy of lives lost that can never be replaced, the numbers loss from the country's population in this appalling event will be replaced in two or three days.

This pace of global population increase cannot be maintained indefinitely. Either birth rates will come down or death rates will go up again, fueled by the fatal cascade of poverty, malnutrition, reduced resistance to disease, and inaccessibility of health care, with resulting epidemic or pandemic. Newly emerging diseases have already begun to reverse the mortality decline that has increased life expectancy in even the world's poorest regions. The AIDS pandemic, an epidemic of epidemics, has now taken more lives than any infectious disease outbreak in modern history.

In a finite world there is obviously a limit to growth but, in fact, no one really knows what number of people is too much, too little, or just right, or how many people the earth can accommodate—its carrying capacity. This remains a dilemma because of the uncertainty of technological progress. Will scientific advances make marginal lands habitable? Can fresh water be brought to arid zones? Can new sources of cheap energy be developed? Can increases in food production be maintained?

Not everyone believes that limiting population growth should be a concern. Part of the disagreement stems from religious ideology. These differences are difficult, if not impossible, to reconcile. The Pope believes, "There is room for all at the banquet of life," and there are no signs of change from this official position by the hierarchy of the Catholic Church. Although Islamic scholars find no proscription of birth control in the Koran, provided methods adopted are reversible, some fundamentalist mullahs adopt a more rigid interpretation. Consequently, in theocratic countries under iron-fisted control by the orthodoxy, such as Afghanistan under the Taliban, for example, only 1–2% of women used some form of birth control, and this was done clandestinely for the sake of self-protection.

When a Commission on Birth Control including theologians and lay-Catholics recommended liberalizing the church's position on contraception, and was disregarded, many Catholics throughout the world were dismayed. First appointed by Pope John XXIII, The Pontifical Commission on Population, Family and Birth had purposely stayed away from the more controversial subjects of abortion and surgical sterilization, believing that this would give more weight to their recommendation that the church liberalize its position and accept the oral contraceptive pill as a sanctioned method of contraception. Commission members believed that the intractable position of John's successor, Pope Paul VI, revealed in the encyclical *Humanae Vitae*, was wrong for Catholic couples and was damaging to the church.

My wife and I were invited to a meeting of the Christian Family Movement, convened after publication of the encyclical. The one other guest couple was Sue and Ansley Coale. Ansley was then the director of Princeton's Office of Population Research. His co-authored article on the relationship between population growth and economic development in Mexico had sparked much of the interest in and attention to population size and growth. The purpose of the meeting, at which we were to be resource persons on technical matters, was to determine what further steps devoted lay-Catholics could take to influence the thinking at the Vatican. Pat Crowley of Chicago, who had been a member of the commission, and his wife Patty, extended our invitations. Eminent and devoted Catholics, with close ties to Church leaders in the United States, they felt greatly honored when Pat was named to the commission, but then felt betrayed when its work was ignored. Pat told me that after the commission submitted its report, the members never had further word from the Vatican and were stunned to read *Humanae Vitae* when it was made public.

The meeting of the Christian Family Movement, an international organization of Catholic couples over which the Crowleys presided, was held in a chateau built on the site of an eleventh century monastery founded by Saint Bernard in La Prée, a small village in the Loire Valley in France. My primary role was to explain the status of modern contraception and in particular the scientific understanding of the pill's mechanism of action. Upon arrival at La Prée after a daylong bus ride from Orly airport, we soon learned of the anguish many of the participants suffered because of the conflict with their church. A Latin American couple told me that in spite of the Vatican's position, in impoverished villages parish priests who were close to the people and their suffering were recommending the pill in confessional booths. A surgeon from Manila sobbed when he explained that he has to find an excuse to do a full hysterectomy when a woman pleads for the simple but illegal tubal ligation operation for sterilization.

Although the Vatican usually leads organized opposition to contraception, other orthodox religions also reject birth control. In the United States, radical fundamentalist Protestant denominations, frequently led by telegenic pastors, tend to be the most vocal, citing the biblical command, "be fruitful and multiply." That may have been good advice for the Garden of Eden when human population density was two per square Earth.

Hardline biologists write about rapid population growth in terms with shock impact: "the population explosion" or "the population bomb." I am also a biologist, but I don't care for these military metaphors. I'm concerned about population because we need to be able to feed, house, educate, and provide health care for all people. To achieve this without degrading the human habitat or upsetting the earth's fragile biosphere, we cannot disregard the consequences of rapid population growth.

The impact of human population on the earth and its resources depends not only on how many people there are, but also on what they do. As standards of living are raised, expectations and demands increase. Like high rates of population growth, overconsumption cannot go on indefinitely. We hear illustrative comparisons but tend to shrug them off and brush them aside. During a lifetime, each child raised in the United States will utilize 20 times as much of the earth's resources as a child raised in India and create 17 times as much waste and pollution. The United States needs as much oil annually for commercial energy use as China and India combined, countries that are home to more than one-third of the world's people. With less than 5% of the world's population, the United States is responsible for 23% of the world's carbon emission, a major factor in global climate change.

As standards of living rise in the rest of the world, these proportions will change, not because Americans will become more energy frugal and environmentally responsible, but because, with growing global affluence, the total demand for and utilization of the earth's resources will rise along with a concomitant increase in wastes and pollution. Hopefully, both Americans and other increasingly affluent people will become more environmentally responsible if given clear guidance by opinion leaders.

The last half of the twentieth century broke all growth records. The world's population increased from 2.5 billion in 1950 to 6 billion. Since we're not making or discovering new land in our finite world, this inevitably led to greater population density. Population density went from an average of 19 persons per square mile to 46—an eye-catching but meaningless statistic. If we don't know what number is ideal for world population size, we certainly can't say what's right for population density. When you think about places with teeming populations, India, China, and Bangladesh come to mind, but, in fact, countries with the highest population density include the lands of tulips, endive, and chocolate bars—Holland, Belgium, and Switzerland—known for their orderliness, cleanliness, and prosperity. Rich and litter-free Singapore has just about the highest population density among nations—eight times that of impoverished Bangladesh. The Netherlands has a population density of 466 persons per square mile. This is 10 times the global average. Yet, most would agree that the Dutch have a wonderful country to live in, and a constant flow of immigrants yearns to join them. So, numbers count, but so do human activities and behavior.

The notion that the world's population expansion is over is wrong; it still has a long way to go. Growth will continue in the early part of the twenty-first century at the rate of nearly 1 billion per decade before the growth rate starts to slow down. Demographers project that as many people will be added to the world's population in the next 50 years as were added in the last 50.

Projections are not predictions. The former is a product of scientific analysis; the latter is the work of soothsayers or fortune cookies. Short term projections of population growth have proven to be remarkably reliable. They are based on national census figures reported to the United Nations, birth and death rates, age structure of a population, age of marriage, and other factors demographers have found to influence population growth. Projections are always reliable over a 5–10 year period, growing less so after that. Adjustments with the passage of time are needed as new information on these factors becomes available. These changes, sometimes discounted by critics as corrections of last year's "best guess," are actually the fine tuning of projections with up-to-date facts.

Current information indicates that if high fertility rates are continued, the world would have 6 billion additional people before stabilization is achieved at the end of the twenty-first century. Following the pattern of recent decades, almost all of this growth (97%) will take place in the countries of the developing world. Over the course of the 1990s, for example, the population of developing countries increased by almost 1 billion, while the population of the industrialized countries grew by merely 40 million or so. The countries of Asia had 3 billion people in 1990. Projected to double this century, Asia then would have to accommodate as many people as there are in the entire world today. Sub-Saharan Africa would experience by far the largest relative growth: a fivefold increase from just over 600 million to almost 3 billion, in spite of the tragic toll of AIDS in some countries. The smallest of the less-developed regions, Latin America, is expected to double its population to about 1 billion during the century. These projections are out to a hundred years, based on currently available information. Circumstances could change. Projections to a closer horizon are more precise. If fertility rates continue to decline in the next decade, an estimated world population between 9 and 10 billion by 2050 is the most likely number, agreed upon by different analysts.

These are the facts and numbers. I do not present them to startle you; that's just the way it is. Some population comparisons are calculated simply for their shock effect. For example, you sometimes read that more people are living today than all previous generations in human history combined. That may be true, but I don't really know what to make of this except, gee whiz. There are also calculations about the future that are "gee whiz" statistics. One of my favorites is what would happen if the human population were to grow at the same rate in the next 10,000 years as it did in the last 10 millennia. The population of the earth would be 6 trillion, and each person would be allotted 10 square meters of space over the entire earth's surface. Closer to real time is the calculation that if the present annual growth rate of 1.65% (a rate that doubles the population every 42 years) were to continue for another century and a half, the population would reach 60 billion, and if it continued unchanged beyond that, the 6 trillion level would be reached a few hundred years later. I doubt that anyone, including their creators, takes these numbers seriously; they serve as a wake-up call that there are limits to growth.

Reality is that the adult world of our grandchildren will have a global population size 3–4 billion higher than today's, and it will still be growing. This is the result of fertility in some countries as high as five or more children per woman and the legacy of even higher birth rates in the recent past.

Over most of human history countries with high birth rates also had almost matching death rates, so that populations remained stable or growth tended to be slow. When this gets out of step and death rates fall while birth rates remain high, population growth soars. This is what happened in the world's poorer regions after World War II. The difference between annual additions to world population (births) and losses (deaths) climbed from roughly 500 million net additions during the 1950s, to 800 million during the 1980s, reaching nearly a billion per decade in the 1990s. This is the level of growth that is continuing into the twenty-first century.

World War II left much of the world in desperate need. Harry S. Truman in his inaugural address after his surprise victory in the 1948 presidential election promised "a bold new program for making available the benefits of our scientific advances to relieve the suffering of the world's impoverished people." This was the announcement of the historical Point Four program which, over the decades, transformed into the U.S. Agency for International Development (U.S. AID). Truman's pledge has been kept by every postwar American administration. The advances of Western industry and science—food production and distribution, antibiotics, public health measures—were provided to the new countries of the postcolonial world.

There is a story, legendary among international health workers, that as the Second World War ended, one shipload of DDT in Colombo, Ceylon (now Sri Lanka) reduced infant death rates by 50%. Malaria was the major cause of infant mortality at that time and simply spraying DDT controlled the mosquito vector of the disease. But the transfer of birth control practice required changes in culture and tradition that proved to be much more intractable. Nevertheless, after a period of lagging behind the decline in death rates, birth rates, too, began to decline. This is called the demographic transition—from high death rates and high birth rates to low death rates and low birth rates.

The transition of the last half of the twentieth century began in East Asia, starting with Japan, Taiwan, South Korea, and the People's Republic of China. Less complicated than talking about death rates, birth rates, and growth rates, another way to describe what happened is in terms of the total fertility rate (TFR), the average number of children born per woman. In East Asia in 1960 the TFR was 5.6. By 2000 it was 1.8. This is below the level of fertility at which each couple, on the average, replaces itself. Theoretically, this would be an even 2, but considering that some couples are infertile or choose to remain childless, a slight upward adjustment for an entire population is necessary, so a fertility rate of 2.1 is the replacement level. The U.N. has recently recommended that the replacement level be lowered somewhat because of advances in child survival and life expectancy. A large component of the dramatic decline in East Asia was in China, the world's most populous nation, but the fertility rates of other countries of the Pacific rim have declined equally or even more. The TFRs of China, Taiwan, North Korea and South Korea, Japan, Singapore, and Hong Kong are all below replacement level.

The Japanese experience is unusual because of the rapidity with which birth rates declined after a post-World War II baby boom and because of its dependency on abortion to reduce the rate of births. For many years, more than half of pregnancies in Japan were terminated before full term. Why and when Japan legalized abortion is an interesting story. After Imperialist Japan had been defeated, the civilian population was left in desperate circumstances. There was little food, a great shortage of housing, and massive unemployment. The post-war Prime Minister Shigeru Yoshida, who was to lead Japan out of the postwar rubble, believed that rapid population growth would impede economic development, so he lent his support to a change in the laws that would make abortion legal. Legal or not, abortion had become a common practice because families were unwilling to have children they could not afford. Backed by a coalition of socialist members who were eager to advance women's reproductive health and conservative members thinking in macroeconomic terms, the Japanese Diet passed the Eugenics Protection Law of 1948 that legalized abortion. The language was not pretty, particularly at a time when the world was stunned by the disclosure of Nazi crimes in the name of eugenics. The stated purpose of the Japanese Law was, "to prevent the birth of eugenically inferior offspring, and to protect maternal health and life." In fact, its intent was to replace back-alley abortions with medically safe procedures done by trained personnel.

The passage of the Eugenics Protection Law would not have been possible without the endorsement of General Douglas MacArthur, the supreme commander of the American Occupation Forces. His archived papers record that he agreed with the argument that rapid population growth would impede recovery efforts, and this probably was the major factor that determined his decision. But there is another element to this story, told to me by the late Professor Minoru Tachi, a distinguished Japanese demographer who was director of Tokyo's Population Problem Research Institute, that helps to explain the general's decision. After the war, the Japanese military and civilians who had been sent to Manchuria and other conquered territories on the mainland were returned to Japan. In retribution for the behavior of Japanese troops in China, particularly the atrocities in Nanking, Manchurian and Chinese soldiers assaulted and raped many women who were part of the exodus, so that among the steady stream of repatriated Japanese a significant number of women returned to Japan in an early stage of pregnancy. It was not unusual for them to resort to abortion, even though it was then illegal. Their plight elicited the sympathy of American women living in Japan with their husbands in the occupation forces. Consequently, the Officer's Wives Club petitioned General MacArthur to throw his support behind the Eugenics Protection Law. That may have clinched the deal for the otherwise socially conservative MacArthur, who had presidential aspirations at that time.

In subsequent years, legal surgical abortion became an important part of the income of gynecologists in Japan, where the percentage of physicians who are gynecologists is the highest in the world. By 1960, fees collected for legal abortions accounted for more than 10% of the private practice income of Japanese specialists in gynecology. Consequently, when the oral contraceptive pill was introduced in the United States and elsewhere in 1960, its approval in Japan was not only a medical decision but also a medical-economic issue. The situation was complicated by the fact that Japan in those years did not enforce its prescription drug rules so that pharmacies could distribute the pill directly, without income-generating office visits to doctors being involved.

This dilemma was explained to me by the then-professor of obstetrics and gynecology of the prestigious Tokyo University, when my wife and I traveled to Japan in 1961. I was on a lecture tour at universities throughout the country. (It was also our honeymoon.) Because the decision on the pill was in the hands of an advisory committee of 11 doctors that included three obstetrician/gynecologists, it seemed unlikely that governmental approval of the pill would be made quickly. Professor Kobayashi, the royal obstetrician who had delivered the son of the crown prince (now Emperor Akihito), was an influential member of the Special Committee for Establishing Standards for Oral Contraceptive Drugs. Initially, the committee did not act or even convene because the experience with oral contraceptives in Japan was extremely limited by the time the first pill, Enovid, was introduced in the United States. The Japanese licensee for Enovid filed an application for drug registration in 1960, presenting data on only 140 cases in which the product had been used for contraception (the drug had already been registered for various gynecological uses). Later, after more information on its use in Japan was assembled, the committee continued its opposition, justified on the basis of uncertainties about cancer risk for Japanese women. With the passing of years, when these doubts were allayed, the concern shifted to other issues such as the pill's possible role in encouraging promiscuity, or the absence of protection against sexually transmitted diseases. Ultimately, it was not until 1999 that approval was signed and Japanese women were finally given access to the contraceptive method that had become so widespread throughout the world.

I have great admiration for my Japanese colleagues and feel greatly honored to have been elected as an honorary member of the Japan Society of Obstetrics and Gynecology. I report these circumstances not in criticism but for the sake of historical accuracy. A recent book on the subject, *Abortion Before Birth Control: The Politics of Reproduction in Postwar Japan,* by Tiana Norgren of Columbia University, presents a detailed historical account of these events.

Another region where abortion was used in place of contraception was the Soviet Union before its fall. There, in the state-controlled economy, it was a macroeconomic decision not to import expensive foreign contraceptives or develop modern contraceptive-manufacturing facilities. By design, apparently, this left the abortion option as women's main recourse to limit fertility. There were locally produced condoms but they were crude and looked like mini-tractor tires. I doubted they could engender consumer confidence or loyalty. During an interview by Barbara Walters on her television program, I showed her a sample that I had brought back from Moscow. She agreed with me.

Shortly before the downfall of the Soviet Union, in 1989, I was invited to a meeting of health officials from most of the Soviet states. Sponsored by the World Health Organization, the meeting took place in Alma Ata (now Almaty) in the Soviet state of Kazakhstan. Here too my role was to talk about the risks and benefits of contraceptive methods. Most of the participants were women doctors. I was amazed when they launched a personal attack on the Central Health Ministry official who was present. When a demographer, Andrey Popov, from Moscow's Academy of Sciences reported that in 1988 there were more than 6,500,000 abortions in the USSR, exceeding the number of live births, and the average number of abortions for a woman in her lifetime was more than 6, the state officials were shocked. They turned their wrath on the Health Ministry doctor. "It is your fault," they accused, "that our women do not have contraceptives!" The Estonian representative spoke openly about ignoring the law in order to help her patients smuggle in IUDs from Finland. After observing this outburst, so much in contrast to previous visits when it was obvious that the central government's decisions in Moscow were beyond criticism, I knew that the Soviet Union was destined to break apart before long.

Abortion rates, incidentally, have remained high in the intervening years. In 1999 there were 1695 abortions for every 1000 live births in Russia. Independent Kazakhstan reports 662 for every 1000 live births. This is about double the rate in the United States.

In India, with its present population of 1 billion, change in reproductive behavior has not gone as fast or as far as the Asian countries of the Pacific rim, but fertility has declined significantly. The 1960 level of more than 6 children per woman fell to 3.1 by the year 2000. The optimist says that this is almost three-quarters of the way to replacement. The realist points out that India's current growth rate will double the population before replacement level of fertility is reached, and the age structure will then drive the population size even higher. India will overtake China in population numbers and become the world's most populous country in about 25 years.

When I lived in India in the 1960s, high fertility seemed an unchangeable feature of the country's way of life for the foreseeable future. Scholars argued that high birth rates were deeply imbedded in Indian culture. Families expected many of their children to die. They needed the labor of many hands, parents required surviving children to care for them in their old age, and Hindu fathers needed living sons to pray for their spirits. An Indian husband expected his bride to produce many children, preferably sons. Until she did, her husband's family, with whom she had to live, treated her disdainfully. A barren daughter-in-law had the lowest status in the household, was given the most arduous tasks, and was the last to be allowed to take food for herself at meals. I have seen this behavior not only in village life, but also among India's most educated families.

These attitudes were believed to be deep rooted, particularly in rural India where 80% of the population lived. In spite of this tradition of high fertility, in just one generation, much of rural India joined its urban counterpart in adopting a new norm of lower fertility, along with other changes in lifestyle such as electrification and television. Indian farmers pioneered in accepting new varieties of grain that required nontraditional methods of cultivation. Moreover, their wives and children are now on the Internet and very much computer literate. The rapidity of these changes seems to have taken many academics who study traditional cultures by surprise. Often, I have had the impression that it is not village dwellers who are slow to accept social change, but the anthropologists who study them.

Countries dominated by fundamentalist theocracies do not follow this global trend. Afghanistan under Taliban rule had a small dip in fertility from 6.8 children per woman in 1985 to 6.0, but further decline is likely as women gain more freedom under more moderate leadership. Pakistan's fertility over the same time span has dropped from 6.7 to about 4.6. In Iran, the average has declined from more than 6 to under 4 children per woman. The world's largest Muslim population is in Indonesia. There, fertility is declining year after year, encouraged by a governmental family planning program and will fall to replacement level by 2015 according to present trends. The Arab countries of the Middle East are following the same course. It is not Islam that keeps fertility high. Governments that subjugate women are the cause.

The countries of Latin America and the Caribbean have also had steep falls in fertility from a regional average of 6 children in 1960 to 2.7 in 2000. The large-population countries, including Brazil and Mexico, have participated in this fertility decline. Brazil will reach replacement level in 2005. The equatorial and Amazonian regions of the northeast are lagging behind the drop in fertility in the large southern cities of Rio and Sao Paulo. Mexico's fertility rate is falling, but it is not expected to be at replacement until 2025.

Regions of Africa will continue to have high fertility levels well into the twenty-first century, according to current projections. Sub-Saharan Africa's average has dropped slowly from 6.6 children per woman in 1960 to 5.2 in 2000. The shift to low fertility is limited so far to just a few countries. In 35 African nations fertility rates still average more than 5 children per woman. The most populous African country, Nigeria, has a TFR of 5.3. In North Africa women were averaging 6 children in 1980, but this has now declined to 3.3.

I am frequently asked, "Why worry? Won't population growth come to an end if we simply wait for these fertility rates to keep falling until they reach replacement levels?" It is unrealistic to think that fertility can continue the rapid decline of the past 30 years. But even if fertility were to immediately decline throughout the world so that starting now, each couple had just 2 children to replace itself, global population would continue to grow for many years because of the young age structure of countries with a recent history of high fertility. The number of children per couple may be smaller, but there would be more couples having children. This creates a momentum of growth that cannot be abruptly halted. It's like trying to stop a fast-moving supertanker. Growth could be slowed only if the present young generation delays marriage and child-bearing and then does not have enough children to replace itself. But that's not a likely scenario under voluntary circumstances.

With more and more young people coming into the reproductive age, even 2 children per couple would continue to cause an increase in total population size. In the rich countries of North America, Europe, and Japan, less than 20% of the population is under 15 years old. In Mexico the percentage is about 40%. In sub-Saharan Africa 45% of the population is under the age of 15. In many Arab or Muslim countries it is as high as 50%. It is inevitable that record numbers will enter their childbearing years over the next decade or two, mostly in the world's poorest regions.

The largest generation in history stands on the threshold of adulthood. Some 800 million are teenagers. This is one-seventh of the world's population; the choices they make will have a profound impact on the world. As they and their younger sisters and brothers reach childbearing age, their decisions on marriage and childbearing will determine the ultimate size of world population. These decisions will be influenced by the opportunities we provide for them, in education, jobs, and other factors that improve the quality of life.

Based on the expected fertility of people already born, the momentum of population growth ensures that the world of 2015 will have more than 7 billion people, and by 2025 world's population will exceed 8 billion. Growth will continue beyond then. Both the United Nations and the U.S. Census Bureau project that by 2050 we will have a world population of 9.3 billion, a number more than half again as large as today's total. As I pointed out earlier, we'll add as many inhabitants to our planet in the next 50 years as we did in the record setting half-century just past.

Population growth depends not only on birth rates, but also on death rates. Looking ahead, decreases or increases in key rates of mortality will influence overall population growth rates. A critical barometer is the infant mortality rate, the number of infants that do not survive the first year of their lives. The highest infant mortality rates are found in Africa, where the average is 92 deaths per 1000 babies born. In many countries in the region the rate exceeds 100, reaching as high as 169 per 1000 in Sierra Leone. In Africa's poorest countries, as many as 20% of children do not reach their fifth birthday.

Compare this to the world's more affluent countries. In high-income countries the infant mortality rate is 6 per 1000, and survival to age five can be expected for more than 99% of newborns. These comparisons can be added to the list of unacceptable differences in health statistics between rich and poor countries. We would all like to see this gap closed. Yet, it is unrealistic to talk about health equity between countries that spend annually more that $3800 per capita on health, such as the United States, or Canada where the national health service spends almost $2000 per person, and countries that budget $6 a year per person, the average for sub-Saharan Africa. Even this pitifully small allocation of national budgets is spent mostly for hospitals in the big cities, with little going to the rural areas where most of the people live.

On the brighter side, a big international push to extend childhood immunization is succeeding in some regions and is beginning to reach into countries with the highest infant and child mortality rates. I am optimistic about the chances for success of this effort and believe it will make major progress in reducing infant and child mortality. Even in the face of political strife and violence, the programs are moving forward. In some countries insurgency groups and government forces have actually declared periods of tranquility so that vaccination teams could reach children. Recently, I saw a dramatic photo of two young women nurses, members of a revolutionary group in El Salvador, with AK-47s slung casually over their shoulders while they immunize small children in a remote village. That has to give you hope for the human spirit.

Vaccination programs have now eliminated polio from the Western Hemisphere and China. Globally, the number of reported cases fell more than 90% between 1988 and 2000. Comprehensive childhood immunization programs can succeed; the technology is available and the determination to do it appears to be strengthening. This will probably be the major factor in the coming years to reduce death rates and increase longevity in developing countries. It can succeed if the world can be kept free of war and the turmoil that causes millions of children to become homeless refugees.

We must face the fact that new killer diseases like AIDS are a constant threat to take away the gains made in reducing the burden of illness. The AIDS epidemic is one of the great tragedies in the history of infectious diseases. It takes the lives of infants and adults, and since the majority of victims are young adults, it leaves behind many orphaned children, still too young to take care of themselves.

All told, more than 50 million people had been infected with the AIDS-causing human immunodeficiency virus (HIV) by the end of 2000. Since its appearance in the 1970s, more than 20 million have died from AIDS, and at least 35 million adults and children are living with the HIV infection. The full picture, however, may be worse, because diagnostic facilities worldwide are limited, and there is a reluctance to report the true number of cases in many countries.

Although none of the world's geographic regions has been spared, Africa, where the epidemic began, has been the hardest hit. In some

African countries there is no family left untouched by the disease. More than 90% of all cases and 95% of AIDS deaths have occurred in the developing world, mostly among young adults and increasingly in women. In recent years, the upsurge in infections that are occurring in Asia, where population size is so large, is adding substantially to the total number and the rate of spread of the disease.

Not only birth rates and death rates influence the world's demographic future. Age structure is important, as well. As the world's population gets larger, it is getting both younger and older. What I mean by this seeming paradox is that the proportions of both older people and children under 15 years are increasing. As I mentioned above, with the beginning of the new century, nearly 1 of every 3 persons is under 15; 800 million are teenagers. For older people, life expectancy is increasing as mortality has decreased even at the oldest ages. Experts on mortality believe that in some countries around the world people can expect to live roughly 20 years longer than their parents or their grandparents.

The traditional age structure of the human population is changing. For centuries, it could be depicted as a pyramid with a wide base representing large numbers of babies born, quickly narrowing because many died in early childhood, and rising to a point depicting few survivors past the age of 65. Now, in the United States, the peak has risen to 85 or higher. Life expectancy at birth has risen to 80.2 for females and 73.5 for males. With advancing age, the elderly are maintaining a participatory role in community affairs and other measures of an active life. The percentage of Americans 65 and older has risen from approximately 4% in 1900 to more than 12% in 2000 and is projected to reach nearly 20% by 2030. Population aging is a global phenomenon. The number of persons worldwide aged 60 years or older was estimated to be nearly 600 million in 2000 and is projected to grow to almost 2 billion by 2050. The older population itself is aging. In the United States the oldest of the old (80 years or older) now make up 11% of the population 60 years or older. In fact, this is the fastest-growing segment of the older population. By 2050, 19% of the older population will be 80 and older.

This achievement is laudable. As Martha Ritche, a former director of the U.S. Census Bureau, explained to me not long ago, "How else can you characterize adding 20 years to healthful life expectancy?" There are solid studies on the quality of life with aging, and these show that it is, indeed, extra years being added to enjoyable living, rather than simply prolonging the painful period of dying.

I heard a seminar on this subject recently by economist Linda Martin, president of the Population Council. The researchers asked questions such as "Are you able to dress or bathe without assistance?" in order to identify change in motor function as the elderly grew older. I suggest that soon the question will be, "Do you still play singles, or have you switched to doubles?" As I watch the octogenarian tennis games in Woods Hole each summer, that question seems more apropos to gage the lifestyle of today's elderly. The quality of play proves that in tennis, it's not how hard you hit it, but where you hit it!

But this changing age structure is not without complications. Social security systems were established when young workers could be expected to live only a few years beyond 65. Now, these systems need to find ways to remain financially viable as the population they support rises and the population that pays into the pension plans dwindles. Economists write about the "dependency ratio" that describes the percentage of the population working to support the nonworking. The dependent groups are people over 65 and those under 15. With people living longer, productive lives, and young people rarely contributing to the adult economy before they have finished their education, there is a new demographic reality influencing dependency ratios.

Not only is there a change in how long people are living, there is also a change in where they choose to live. For the first time in human history, the world's population is about to become predominantly urban, not rural. Early in the twenty-first century, rural dwellers will be in the minority. By 2025 the urban share of the population may exceed 60%. This urban expansion has been fueled in part by massive population shifts from rural to urban areas and by preferential cross-border immigration to cities in search of job opportunities. Since 1950, the urban population of industrialized countries has nearly doubled. In the developing world, although there are regional differences, it has swelled five times. Seventy-five percent of the population of Latin America and the Caribbean is urban. More than a third of the Asian population is now urban, compared to just 20% a few decades ago. In Africa, a traditionally rural population is now 40% urban.

The United States has experienced a historic transfer of population from farm to city throughout the latter half of the twentieth century, so that only a small portion of the population is engaged in agriculture.

Fewer than 5 million workers are employed in agriculture, out of a total civilian labor force of more than 140 million. Agriculture contributes but 2% to the gross domestic product.

Many cities have reached gigantic proportions, making it virtually impossible for municipalities to keep ahead of the demand for infrastructure and services. In numerous developing country cities, housing, roads, health care, educational facilities, and the provision of safe drinking water and sanitation have not kept up with the rising tide of urban dwellers. In places such as Calcutta or Mumbai, city planners have actually drawn up plans to build new adjacent cities rather than try to upgrade infrastructure in the present metropolitan areas. Mexico City has to pump almost all of the fresh water for its 10 million inhabitants from sea-level sources to its mile-high location. It is a daunting challenge. Yet over the next decade the population is expected to grow by another 3 million.

I recently participated in a government-sponsored symposium in Mexico City, along with local officials concerned with consequences of population growth. We had discussions about air pollution and fresh water needs, as was predictable, but I was surprised that urbanization was emphasized by one of the senior government officials. He could see no solution to unsustainable urban growth in Mexico without a turn to the government controlling internal migration by issuing permits for where people are permitted to reside.

Many unemployed or unskilled marginally employed people end up in slums and squatter communities, undernourished and chronically sick. In some cities that we enjoy visiting as tourists—Delhi or Cairo, for example—the unseen majority of people live in slums. Hundreds of thousands more end each day on the streets, where they find shelter in makeshift shacks fashioned from what they can find. As a foreigner living in New Delhi, it is a shaking experience to realize that anything you discard, a cardboard box or a large crate, can become the only dwelling for a homeless family. While it is true that you can find homeless people even in Sweden's social democracy, where it takes some ingenuity to slip out of the government-provided safety net, or on the streets of New York City in spite of its municipal shelters, there is no comparison in the scale or magnitude found in the world's poorest cities.

The urban area of Delhi grew 13-fold in the twentieth century; it has absorbed more than 100 villages. In picturesque Bahia, Brazil, the city of Salvador, once nestled compactly along the shore of the Bay of All Saints, now spreads both up and down the ocean shoreline and inland to the once-remote airport. The population has grown from less than 200,000 in the 1960s to more than 3 million. The final stretch of the airport road has always been lined with thick bamboo trees (or are they bushes?) that now arch over the roadway at an impressive height. During my last visit, I was saddened to learn that in order to widen the road to accommodate the increase in traffic, the bamboo border will have to be cut down. Who would have thought that those majestic bamboos would be chopped away before having a chance for their once-in-a-100-year blooming! I was looking forward to it.

Today, Los Angeles, New York, London, and Tokyo figure prominently on the list of the world's largest cities. Given current rates of urban growth, by 2025 the world's megacities will all be in developing countries. As the great shift from rural life continues, people unaccustomed to urban dwelling are creating mega-cities of 10–20 million around the globe. Crime, pollution, slums, and poverty are urban realities that are magnified as cities grow to proportions never before imaginable.

Consider these numbers. Lagos, a city of about 1 million in 1950, will soon be one of the world's top 3, with 25 million inhabitants. That will mean that more than 10% of people living in Africa's most populous country will be crowded into one city, already suffering from inadequate infrastructure and social services. Think about São Paulo or Mexico City, with 19 million. Our southern neighbors in Latin America and the Caribbean will be 80% urban in 2015. Tokyo, at the top of the numbers chart for city size, will undoubtedly accommodate the growth from 27 million to 28 million in the next decade, but will Mumbai go from 17 million to 27 million without deteriorating?

Urbanization will be the major trend in the movement of people in the coming years. Particularly in the poorer countries, this explosive growth will test the capacity of governments to generate jobs and to provide the services, infrastructure, and social supports necessary to sustain livable and stable environments. People will be flocking to cities not only from the countryside, but also from cross-border migration. These days, migrants mainly end up in big cities, not as rural dwellers. If they do come for jobs as fruit pickers or farmhands, it doesn't take long before they move on to the city. Urban centers grow as migrants arrive in industrialized countries like Japan and the European Union where they are needed to relieve labor shortages because of aging populations and low birthrates. Poor countries, where there is already unemployment or underemployment, sometimes receive huge numbers of migrants and refugees, frequently survivors from civil conflict, natural disasters, food shortage, or economic crises. All over the world, there are people on the move. In China alone, one estimate has 100 million people drifting from countryside to city or from town to town.

The globalization of labor markets, droughts and other natural disasters, and political instability will fuel global movement of people. Over the next 15 years, migrants will continue to move to North America primarily from Latin America and East and South Asia, to European Union countries primarily from North Africa, the Middle East, South Asia, and from the post-Communist states of Eastern Europe and Eurasia. Political extremists can be expected to enflame popular sentiments against migrants, protesting the strain on social services and the foreign-ness of new arrivals. This trend is already evident in recent elections.

It is not my intention to create an apocalyptic image of unlivable conditions caused by migrating masses and endless urban blight consisting chiefly of unthinkable slums. Judging from past human experience, I believe that the demographic transition from rural to urban along with city growth fostered by immigration will be manageable issues. There is no question that human migration and urbanization rank high among the volatile situations facing the world today, and the results will not be pretty. Sociologists warn that traditional family and social structures are not prepared to cope with the new conditions, as people move from their traditional homes to mega-cities that are strange to them. Futurists predict ethnic conflict, political reaction against migrants, and the sparking of contentious issues among governments.

The horrendous events of September 11, 2001, awakened us to the vulnerability of large cities to attack by unexpected means. New York, the storied city of the world's most powerful nation, could not be protected from commercial airliners taken over by fanatical terrorists and converted to passenger-carrying guided missiles that destroyed a substantial portion of the financial district of Manhattan Island. While not a migration issue, or a matter of internal ethnic conflict, September 11 illustrates the vulnerability of cities, a threat that always existed but that we appear to be powerless to prevent. London, Paris, Barcelona, Tel Aviv, Munich, Cairo, Luxor, Beirut, Nairobi, Moscow, New Delhi, Srinigar—they, too, have experienced urban vulnerability.

In 2000, the CIA's National Intelligence Council released a study on *Global Trends 2015*. I doubt that when the report was written its authors expected the fulfillment in a matter of months of some of their most ominous warnings. They wrote in December 2000, "Between now and 2015 terrorist tactics will become increasing sophisticated and designed to achieve mass casualties. We expect the trend toward greater lethality in terrorist attacks to continue. . . . Some potential adversaries will seek ways to threaten the US homeland."

Ethnic conflict and mass migration were responsible for one of the great human tragedies of the twentieth century as Hindus and Muslims by the millions were forced to flee their homes after the partition of British India in 1947. The violent events of partition were tragic, with countless lives lost due to religious strife, but the receiving cities, on both sides on the new border, managed to absorb the sudden influxes of large masses of people, even though they were changed abruptly. In Calcutta, untold numbers of refugees were forced to sleep in the street, in railway stations, and in other public places. Bombay had more employment opportunities, so that assimilation of the new migrants went more smoothly. Nevertheless, nearly half of Bombay's population had to settle for life in slums or squatter housing.

When large cities are suddenly forced to absorb large numbers of new inhabitants, housing is one of the most serious problems. Overnight, shanty towns appear constructed of just about anything people can get their hands on. When I lived in New Delhi, the municipality's response was to make unannounced dawn raids with baton-wielding police and bulldozers. The police routed the people out of harm's way, and the bulldozers leveled their homes, burying in the rubble their meager belongings. Needless to say, a new shantytown would appear overnight somewhere nearby.

After learning from these fruitless efforts, Delhi authorities recognized that the success of urban management required regional planning efforts. Assistance was given to shanty dwellers so that they could disperse into the surrounding townships. Other cities in India have followed this example by creating regional planning boards in cooperation with their neighboring townships. Ingenuity has had to play a role.

Decentralization, privatization of services, and community-based support groups all can help sustain the quality of urban life in the face of seemingly impossible conditions.

Planners have developed a number of strategies. Mumbai, for example, has adopted the concept of a twin city to facilitate redistribution of the population. It involves developing a number of small townships, sometimes actually constructing them from the ground up. These communities include chiefly low-income housing for a large segment of the urban population, along with the development of offices and commercial buildings, in order to relieve congestion in the old city and create employment opportunities. Bangkok has invested in improving the living conditions within slum neighborhoods.

The rapid growth of the urban population throughout Mexico City over the past years has made it impossible for urban infrastructure to keep pace with needs. Squatter settlements have mushroomed on the city's periphery, causing the physical limits of the central area to become tightly compressed. Water and sanitation services are neither sufficient nor efficient. I've already mentioned a panel I attended in which a government official of Mexico asserted that he could not see a solution for the growing problems of a rapidly expanding Mexico City population other than greater socialization with stricter government control over the movement of people.

Long term, I believe that Mexico City, like the cities of India, must plan on decentralization of both industry and population. There needs to be a movement of industry out of Mexico City. The people will follow without government mandates, I believe.

On a positive note, there are examples of smooth transition of forced migrants into a new life. I have always been impressed with the way the Finns handled the mass migration when Stalinist Soviet Union snatched a third of their small nation after World War II. The people of Karelia, an estimated 400,000, were forced refugees as they arrived in the remaining regions of Finland. Resources were shared, all Finns made sacrifices, and there were no such things as refugee camps. No generation of Finns had to give up their aspirations and live dependent on international handouts. This is the example of the human spirit that I prefer to envisage rather than the slums or barbed-wire detention camps of displaced persons or refugees.

African cities have the added dilemma of the HIV/AIDS epidemic as their cities grow, fostering conditions for the easier spread of the disease. Urban slum dwellers in Nairobi, for example, have a higher incidence of HIV than the city average. Africa also finds urban growth fueled by growing numbers of people who can no longer gain a secure livelihood in their villages because of environmental degradation. Desertification, deforestation, soil erosion, and drought create environmental refugees who feel they have no alternative but to seek sanctuary elsewhere, however hazardous the attempt. With each new dam construction, either for hydroelectric power or irrigation projects, hundreds of thousands of people are involuntarily displaced from their homes. They end up in cities ill-prepared for their arrival.

City planners, architects, and social service innovators will face giant challenges as the world changes more and more into urban living. Most of the issues I have written about are interrelated. More people require more housing, more food and water, and more energy. As they leave rural areas and congregate in mega-cities, they need infrastructure support that requires huge investments, larger than most of the poorer countries can afford. Twenty million people living in one city create enormous waste and spew out large amounts of atmospheric pollutants. Their exposure to city-made pollutants causes health problems and diseases that stretch the resources of health services.

Not only is the world changing with respect to the numbers of people and where they live, but also in the opportunities for women to live a fulfilling life. For much too long, the world has been populated by two categories of people, one underprivileged, undereducated, frequently underfed, and certainly inadequately cared for by health services. The rest are men. Historic changes are beginning to take place. Although there is still great gender inequity, women are beginning to achieve progress in empowerment, in the ability to fulfill hopes and aspirations, in the global workforce, and even in political leadership. Opportunities that John D. Rockefeller 3rd had in mind when he spoke at the 1974 population conference in Bucharest are beginning to open for women in many countries. He would have been pleased to attend a recent panel discussion at the Council on Foreign Relations chaired by his niece Peggy Dulany, in which the panelists were the executive director of UNICEF, the executive director of the U.N. World Food Program, the director-general of the World Health Organization, the executive director of UNFPA, and the U.N. high commissioner for Human Rights—all women.

In spite of this progress, in the United States and elsewhere around the industrialized world, much remains to be done toward gender equality, but the greatest need for improving the status of women is in the female-subjugating, son-preferring cultures of the developing world. Girls and women are hardly given the opportunity to learn to read and write. Around the world, more than 130 million children are not attending school; two-thirds are girls. In Pakistan, only 17% of rural girls complete primary school education. When the Taliban ruled Afghanistan, their mullahs decreed that it was a crime according to Koranic law to educate girls. This interpretation of the teachings of the Koran is a distortion, but it is likely to resurface if similar fundamentalist regimes come to power in other Muslim theocracies.

In other countries the education of girls is neglected because of cultural patterns that favor sons. More than boys, girls are burdened with household responsibilities such as caring for younger siblings, housework, and menial tasks that their parents decide are adequate reasons to keep them from attending school.

Accompanied by my wife, I once visited an agricultural research farm in Gujarat, India, where cows and water buffaloes were being bred for high milk yield. I was impressed by the science that produced the magnificent animals that were paraded before us. Some were record producers of dairy products. But what caught our attention was a small girl of about 10 or 11, whose job it was to trail the animals to gather up the steaming cow dung and shape it into patties. Left out in the sun to dry, cow-dung patties would later be used for fuel or to insulate the primitive huts in which families lived. Covered to her elbows in cow dung and trying to brush from her face the inevitable swarm of flies was part of her daily existence. Of course, she didn't go to school with her brothers.

Years later I saw a striking photograph of a Bengali woman in Bangladesh, old beyond her years, bent, forlorn, and tired, captured by the camera's lens as she looked up from her work of shaping dung with a seemingly endless field of patties laid out behind her, apparently the product of her day's labor. I thought of the little girl in Gujarat and wondered if her life had brought more meaning and chance for fulfillment.

During another trip with my wife and two high-school age daughters, we visited a village in the neighboring state of Madhya Pradesh. We were being shown a demonstration nutrition program that provided supplementary food for underweight children. Jennifer asked how many of the children enrolled were boys and how many girls. The clerk bragged about their record keeping, turned to his card files, and proudly reported that he could tell us that three out of four were boys! Our guide, a state health official, confided that even when underweight girls were enrolled, the nutritional cookies allotted to them were taken home to be shared with their brothers.

The children of India were endlessly fascinating, but we discovered on that trip that we were equally intriguing to them. Our car suffered a broken fan belt on the road to Gwalior. When our driver went in search of a replacement, we were surrounded by curious children, boys and girls. They were intrigued by the braces that both Jennifer and Laura were sporting on their teeth. "What are those?" they asked. They were highly amused by my light-hearted reply. "Those are bangles for the teeth!"

Anyone who has traveled through rural India or Africa has seen graceful young girls who should be in school, walking along a roadside balancing on their heads or hips a packet of twigs or a brass vessel filled with water. As a Rockefeller Foundation officer, in cooperation with state officials of Madhya Pradesh, I helped plan a program aimed at extending education for young girls. An economist attached to the Indian Embassy in Washington had first proposed the idea. In a village not far from the ill-fated city of Bhopal, families or the village itself would be paid a small stipend for every year beyond the prevailing term that young girls were allowed to stay in school. The idea was to offset the family costs of losing their young daughters to the classroom and to give fathers the idea that there is some value to having daughters. It was one of my biggest disappointments in foundation work that this project was never funded and implemented. I think that now, almost 20 years later, in addition to changing the lives of some fortunate youngsters, it could have been an excellent demonstration of the value of educating girls. Perhaps it was an idea that was ahead of its time.

At about that time my friend Muhammad Yunus of Chittagong, Bangladesh, had a better idea that took off like a rocket. Muhammad may be the world's most successful banker, but I doubt if he has ever been invited to Davos to listen to Alan Greenspan. In 1978 Dr. Yunus, a university professor, started a program aimed at helping impoverished families, primarily women. Here is the way it worked: Defying the usual banking rules, he lent them money without collateral so they could start small enterprises like weaving, roadside vegetable stands, or rice processing. The women would form small groups with an agreement of mutual liability, and the group would pay from its profits if one individual member defaulted.

Loans could be arranged in minutes and sometimes were paid back the same day. A woman could borrow enough money in the morning to buy merchandise for a roadside stand selling spices. In the evening she would return what she borrowed, keep the profit to feed her family, and repeat the process the next day. By 1979, when I first met Yunus, he could report that his clients had a repayment rate of 99%. It was a no-brainer for us at the Rockefeller Foundation to support his innovative Grameen Bank and to help others around the world develop similar micro-credit plans. The list of nongovernmental organizations that were quick to recognize the value of micro-credit to help women start micro-enterprises is impressive: Save the Children Foundation; Catholic Relief Services, and American Jewish World Services, to name a few. In a vote of confidence, the World Bank has set aside $200 million for micro-credit programs.

Meanwhile, the Grameen Bank and many of its look-alikes grew to amazing size and loan volume. After 20 years, the original bank was able to sell $163 million in bonds to regular commercial banks in Bangladesh and thereby cut free from dependence on the donor agencies that helped Yunus get started. He is a man of great vision and even greater expectations. His hope is that his micro-credit scheme will reach 100 million of the world's poorest families, especially the women of these families, by 2005. Yunus likes to refer to the global micro-credit network as the World Bank for the poor. When Yunus talks, people listen. The buzzword in the investment world of rich countries during the past decade has been e-commerce. Most of the world's poor people may never have heard of e-commerce, but they do know about micro-credit.

The world is changing. It is becoming more urban than rural, equity for women is recognized as a strategy to reduce poverty, and apart from countries affected by AIDS, people are living longer. In his perceptive book, *The Lexus and the Olive Tree*, Thomas Friedman explains why, in the world of globalization of economics and communications, many changes are irreversible. For the same reasons, the demographic transition to low mortality and low fertility is not reversible. In spite of the efforts of some fundamentalist and reactionary elements in all countries, including the United States, to reestablish female subjugation, it won't happen. Afterthought apologies notwithstanding, rational people scorn the intemperate remarks of Jerry Falwell and Pat Robertson that modern feminism is part of the package of "sins" for which the United States was punished on September 11, 2001.

Everywhere, women can "sign on" and expand their borders beyond the male-dominated limits on education and freedom imposed by leaders of their countries and communities. They will not allow the progress of recent years to be taken away from them. They will not give up the advances they have made in having a voice in decisions about their own fertility and family size.

In Catholic Brazil, I saw a poster in CEPARH, a women's health center. It is a message that women around the world understand. The poster depicted a beautiful, tasteful nativity scene. It read, "Mary had but one child and he changed the world."

2

Vulnerable Links in the Chain of Reproductive Events

Think of the entire human presence on earth (about 350,000 years) as a 24-hour day. Then the last 5000 years of recorded history becomes but a few minutes, and the time during which people have been able to exert willful control over their fertility is a flashing millisecond during *Homo sapiens'* day on earth.

In a world of 6 billion people, there are more than 1 billion couples of reproductive age that have coitus an estimated 110 billion times a year, resulting in the fertilization of about 300 million human eggs. Some 100 million of these fertilized eggs simply pass out unnoticed with the menstrual flow. Seventy million that do connect to the mother's uterus and start to develop into embryo or fetus end up as miscarriages or are electively aborted. The remaining fertilized eggs, roughly 130 million, proceed through the entire 9 months of pregnancy and result in newborn babies.

The human reproductive system is basically unchanged from that of our original *Homo sapiens* ancestors, but the typical pattern of a woman's reproductive years has changed. Culture, not biology, ended the eons of incessant reproduction when sexually mature women were pregnant or lactating almost constantly until an early death. Women now have an occasional pregnancy followed by some months of breast-feeding. Consequently, they spend most of the years between menarche and menopause using some means of birth control and menstruating each month. Modern lifestyles and family life have moved the human female from the era of reproduction to the era of contraception and menstruation. This may have been the most important social movement of the twentieth century for women.

The contraceptive methods couples use now are such recent arrivals that they would not even appear as a blip on the radar scan of human history. The successful struggle for women's right to vote came far earlier in history than the right of women to control their own reproduction. When pioneering feminist Susan B. Anthony in 1887 challenged her critics with the provocative question, "are women persons?" she could not have known anything about the safe period or the biology of the menstrual cycle. This was not because of a deficiency in her education, but because science and medicine had not progressed to that stage. The scientific knowledge that led to the pill, for example, is a product of hormone research done in the second half of the twentieth century. Earlier in the 1900s, medical schools were still teaching that a woman's period was a sign that she had just ovulated, an idea erroneously taken from observing the reproductive behavior of some animals. Many contemporary women still do not have accurate information about their own reproductive process.

After giving a guest lecture at Wellesley College, I was approached by a polite young woman who looked like she might be a freshman or sophomore. "Excuse me, professor," she said, "I always heard that the time you have to be careful is just after menstruation because that's when you ovulate. You said it was in the middle of the month. Is that true?" I'm glad I had a chance to straighten out the facts for her before she spent any more years at the Wellesley-Cambridge social scene. And what about the rest of the world? Remember the infertility clinic in rural India I wrote about in the introduction? Dr. Southam and I were amazed at the number of couples for whom the inability to conceive was a serious problem, but who had no understanding of the optimal time for a successful conception.

History and anthropology have many examples of the misunderstanding of how the human reproductive process works. I once shared a panel discussion with the legendary anthropologist Margaret Mead, author of *Coming of Age in Samoa*. After my talk on the history of modern contraception, she told me that Samoans believed that a woman became pregnant by sitting under a banana tree during the full moon. We agreed that she should look into the "with whom" question.

The human reproductive process has a defining feature. Every month from the time of puberty, the woman's body prepares for a possible pregnancy. This is the genetically controlled system that has proved to have the adaptive advantages and survival power that has enabled *Homo sapiens* to go from the original few who evolved from earlier manlike hominoids to the 6 billion plus we number today. Evolution could have mapped out a different plan for human reproduction. For example, many mammals are seasonal breeders. In this system the female's body undergoes preparation for pregnancy just once a year, and behavioral changes in both the male and female make certain that the opportunity to reproduce will not be lost. In other species the female responds to copulation and cervical stimulation by releasing many eggs and preparing the uterus for pregnancy. Because intercourse, ovulation, and the start of pregnancy are all integrated, the system assures high-performance reproduction. Still another strategy might have been the routine birth of a litter-size number of offspring with the expectation that at least one might survive.

The human system is programmed around the monthly development of one egg, ordinarily. For the process to work efficiently, however, it is equally essential that the rest of the woman's reproductive system is prepared to receive the egg and, if it is fertilized, protect it as development begins, physically attach the conceptus to the mother, and maintain it throughout pregnancy and delivery. How this all comes about is clearer now that we understand much about the endocrinology and genetics of reproduction. There is still plenty left for future reproductive scientists to discover, as they look deeper into fundamental mechanisms of the endocrinology of reproduction, discover the involvement of new proteins and genes, and puzzle over still unanswered questions of how embryological cells differentiate. Why did a nose cell become a nose and not an ear?

The reproductive process is a well-organized system of interrelated behavioral and physiological events and anatomical changes that proceed in perfect synchrony under the influence of hormones secreted by the brain, the pituitary gland, and the gonads. The woman's ovaries and the man's testes are central to the process. These sex glands have two vital functions. They produce gametes (eggs or sperm) and they produce the sex hormones. The gametes carry hereditary information from generation to generation by virtue of the union of the male and female genomes. This is the characteristic feature of sexual reproduction. The sex hormones control the secondary sex characteristics that play a supportive role to the gametes.

Biologically, the involvement of the male ends with fertilization; the female goes on to harbor the fertilized egg in a protective and nutritive environment. The entire process is regulated by a series of chemical messengers that reach their destinations through the bloodstream. These chemical messengers control the successive events of egg or sperm development, transport, fertilization, implantation of the fertilized egg in the wall of the uterus, and pregnancy.

This synchronized relay of molecular messages begins in specialized nerve cells in the brain. Sensing the levels of hormones in the bloodstream and responding to external stimuli, at the appropriate time these neurons release small molecules that reach the hypothalamus, a neurosecretory structure at the base of the brain. On receiving the appropriate molecular or electrical message, the hypothalamic cells discharge a small hormone consisting of 10 amino acids: gonadotropin-releasing hormone (GnRH). These polypeptide molecules move into a short, local system of small capillaries that carry them a few centimeters to the pituitary gland. In response, the pituitary discharges two large protein hormones, luteinizing hormone (LH) and follicle-stimulating hormone (FSH), which enter the bloodstream and are carried to the relatively distant sex glands. Because they stimulate the gonads, they are called gonadotropins. They are in the same group of pituitary hormones as the more familiar human growth hormone, thyroid-stimulating hormone, and adrenocorticotropic hormone (ACTH).

In the female LH and FSH participate in unison in stimulating ovarian function. FSH is responsible chiefly for causing the maturation of the ovary's Graffian follicles, which contain the immature eggs in a sheath of primitive nurse cells. In the process, the hormone-secreting cells of the follicle are stimulated to produce increasing amounts of estrogens, and the immature egg is brought to the state of maturation necessary for ovulation. When the estrogen level has reached its peak, levels of the other gonadotropin, LH, also peak and trigger the ovulation process. The mature egg leaves the follicle through a small tear in the outer surface of the ovary, and the empty follicle is transformed into a temporary hormone-secreting organ that produces large amounts of progesterone. This empty follicle is called the corpus luteum, Latin for "yellow body." Because of their effects on sex behavior and secondary sex characteristics, estrogen and progesterone are usually referred to as sex steroid hormones, but they also affect other organs, including bone, muscle, blood, and liver, as well as processes such as carbohydrate metabolism and water retention. The steroid designation refers to their chemical structure.

Next in the molecular relay of reproduction, the steroid hormones stimulate individual cells of the reproductive organs. Upon reaching a target cell, the steroid molecule binds with receptor proteins and the hormone–receptor complex migrates to the nucleus. This hormone–receptor complex activates or inhibits certain genes, altering the cell's program of protein synthesis. In this manner a nonstimulated cell of the uterus, for example, is converted to the stimulated state. Estrogen causes one type of reprogramming of the cell; progesterone causes another.

When scientists began to understand the genetic control of protein synthesis, my friend and colleague Pran Talwar of New Delhi and I were working together in my New York laboratory. We theorized that you should be able to prevent the action of estrogen or progesterone by interfering with the production of a nucleic acid involved in protein synthesis. This proved to be correct, so we went one step further and showed that if you skipped the estrogen or progesterone and treated the uterus with estrogen-induced nucleic acid instead, the uterine cells would respond as if they were hormone treated. This, too, worked in rat and chick experiments, adding to the mounting evidence on the mechanism of action of estrogens and progesterone.

Most of the same molecules play analogous roles in the human male. As in females, integrated processes control both sperm and hormone production by the testis. The hypothalamic and pituitary messengers are the same in both sexes. An important difference is that the patterns of production of the hypothalamic GnRH, the pituitary's gonadotropic hormones, and the gonadal steroids are on a monthly cycle in the female but not in the male. The male does have a daily cycle and even an hourly cycle for the release of some hormones, but this does not play the same vital role that cyclicity over the menstrual month does in the female. The main androgenic sex hormone of the testis is testosterone, although various precursors or metabolites can be found in the body and some have specialized roles in effecting behavior or bodily organs. An enzymatic reaction converts testosterone to the active form that stimulates the man's prostate gland, for example. These androgenic hormones are responsible for the characteristics we recognize as masculine in all species. The mane of the lion, the antlers of the elk, the rooster's comb, and the horns of the ram are all the work of one androgen or another, usually testosterone.

The human ovary receives its supply of eggs early in development. At about the sixth week after fertilization, a small group of stem cells migrate from the inner lining of the embryo's yolk sac into the developing ovary. These stem cells, or oogonia, become the source of all the eggs produced in a lifetime. In the course of embryonic and fetal development, their number increases tremendously through cell division, reaching perhaps 5 million before the multiplication phase ends. However, most of these degenerate during fetal life so that, at birth, the two ovaries of the female infant contain nearly 500,000 primordial follicles, each containing an individual oocyte, the precursors of mature eggs. There will be no more follicles or oocytes added during her lifetime. I refer to this evolutionary adaptation as restriction of the multiplication phase of egg cells. Oddly, most of the eggs and their ovarian follicles are destined for spontaneous degeneration (atresia), a process that starts during fetal life. Atresia continues during childhood and adolescence and throughout the reproductive years. Atresia is the dominant fate of human oocytes. It is only the occasional egg that actually ovulates and has the opportunity to be fertilized—fewer than 500 eggs in a woman's reproductive years. A statistician might say that the number of eggs ovulated in a lifetime is statistically insignificant. A population biologist would probably disagree. Atresia remains a puzzle to scientists. Almost everything about the process except its relentless progress has escaped scientific explanation.

Human reproduction is sexual. In biological terms this means that male and female gametes fuse to create a new genetic constitution carrying hereditary information passed down from the parents. The DNA of the chromosomes contains the entire human genome of 50,000–100,000 genes, about 3% of which are active genes at any given time. At fertilization, the egg contributes a set of 22 autosomes plus an X sex chromosome. The sperm brings a complementary set of 22 autosomes and either an X or a Y sex chromosome. The offspring will be female if the fertilizing sperm carries an X chromosome. Y-bearing sperm produce males. Sexual reproduction is found throughout the animal and plant kingdoms, but other living forms, such as bacteria, viruses, and many plants reproduce differently. Remember watching paramecium reproduce by fission in your high school biology class? That was an example of asexual reproduction.

In sexual reproduction, the genetic sex is determined at fertilization. A fertilized egg is either XX (female) or XY (male), and until the formation of the gonads during embryonic development, chromosomal constitution is the sole manifestation of sex. The sex of an individual is the aggregate of genetic, anatomical, physiological, and behavioral characteristics that are recognized as maleness or femaleness; the differentiation of the gonad into either an ovary or a testis; and the capacity to produce sperm or egg.

One can speak of a male muscular configuration or a female pattern of body fat distribution. Even the chemistry of the blood is sex specific. An individual develops sexuality gradually beginning with the establishment of genetic sex at fertilization, proceeding to the differentiation of the reproductive tract and other familiar secondary sex characteristics, and ultimately involving all of the body including the brain. Consequently, the process of developing sexuality influences attitudes, responses, and other aspects of behavior.

Species that lay huge numbers of eggs, such as the frog, achieve a 50:50 sex ratio among newly hatched tadpoles by the random chance of each egg being fertilized by Y-bearing or X-bearing sperm. Some species have other mechanisms that come into play. A European frog living in the Alps takes advantage of temperature differences to determine whether tadpoles will differentiate as males or females, regardless of genetic sex.

The single human egg has a slightly better chance of being fertilized by a sperm carrying a Y sex chromosome, so that instead of 50:50, the primary sex ratio at fertilization is about 107 males to 100 females. Why this is so, nobody can really say. One theory is that the Y-bearing sperm swims faster than the Y-bearing sperm. The rationale behind this is that the X chromosome is larger than the Y chromosome.

I doubt the first-one-to-get-there theory and believe it has something to do with an active selection of the fertilizing sperm by the egg. During fetal life, as in all other stages of life, there is a slightly higher age-specific mortality rate for males, so that the actual ratio of males to females at birth is about 103 to 100.

Although the genome of the sperm determines sex, the egg is an active participant in the fertilization process. For example, the human egg produces chemical attractants to lure passing sperm to its surface. It also assures that only one sperm fertilizes and blocks others from passing through the egg's outer membrane. This is called the block to polyspermy. This seemingly incidental feature of the reproductive process is, in fact, critical to survival of the species. In the rare cases when the block to polyspermy fails and more than one sperm enters the egg, the resultant polyspermic egg does not survive after a few divisions. A philosopher friend recently told me that he has read of human chimeras that have the DNA makeup that could only result from two sperm having fertilized the same egg. The embryologist in me says it is unlikely, but I will concede that there may be an occasional case that successfully slips by the block to polyspermy and goes on to some stage of development with some cells having one paternal DNA fingerprint and others having another.

Each month, from among the thousands of primary follicles in the ovary, a few start to develop as the circulating FSH levels start to rise. After about 10 days, usually only one dominant follicle continues to flourish and becomes fully mature, ready to release its egg. At midcycle, on approximately the 14th day, ovulation occurs, and the oocyte bursts from the rupture point in a cascade of follicular cells and fluid. Observed and photographed by both scientists and videographers, this critical event in the life cycle resembles the beauty of celestial displays of shooting stars. The released egg is swept away from the surface of the ovary by the undulating open end of the fallopian tube.

The spectacle of ovulation was captured in a wonderful film by Richard Blandau, a famous anatomist from Seattle. Years ago, my daughter's third-grade class visited our laboratory, and I showed them Dr. Blandau's film. For the purpose of the microphotography, the egg, released from the ovary of a rabbit, had been stained blue to make it easier to see and to follow its course. The fascinated children were full of questions. The one I always remember is: "Was the baby rabbit blue?"

At ovulation, the egg contains 46 chromosomes, the normal human complement. Before it is fertilized the number has to be reduced to half. This is achieved by the expulsion of two polar bodies, each carrying a haploid (half) set of chromosomes reducing the genetic material by half, so that the union of an egg with 23 chromosomes and a sperm, also with 23, will produce the normal complement of hereditary material. There is also genetic information in the cytoplasm of the egg. Intracellular organelles called mitochondria contain DNA. This DNA is totally maternal and plays a key role in programming the fertilized egg for the initial steps in development. A tiny portion of a person's genetic information is carried in this mitochondrial DNA.

Fertilization occurs when, around the time of ovulation, sperm ascend to the fallopian tube. Timing is critical. Although sperm can live for several days in the female tract, the released egg is fertilizable for only about 24 hours. The ideal situation for success is when fresh sperm are present in the upper third of the fallopian tube, the arena of fertilization, waiting for the egg to be released. There have been theories proposed, never supported by valid evidence, that one sex or the other is more likely if the sperm is waiting for the egg or vice versa.

Once explained as a simple matter of sperm–egg interaction, fertilization is now understood to be an intricate series of steps that begins when a sperm makes contact with the zona pellucida, a viscous envelope surrounding the egg. By enzymatic action the sperm slices through the zona and makes contact with the egg surface. This initiates a series of functional and structural responses. Sperm–egg contact prompts changes in the zona pellucida that make it impenetrable to additional sperm. In case there are already secondary sperm present in the zona, they are thwarted by alterations in the egg's surface proteins that prevent attachment.

As far as we know, the fertilizing sperm becomes passive at this point, and the egg takes charge. The image of a sperm drilling its way into the passive egg is misleading. Microvilli, tiny fingerlike projections, on the surface membrane of the egg engulf the attached sperm's head and guide it through the outer membrane into the egg's cytoplasm as the sperm tail is detached and left behind. This activates the egg to expel its second polar body, bringing its chromosome number down to the required 23. Even at this point, it is not clear that the egg is fertilized. Within the cytoplasm, the formation of distinct egg and sperm pronuclei unfolds. The pronuclei move together gradually. Then, following structural changes, the maternal and paternal genomes intermingle, and with this event the first cell division of the fertilized egg begins. After 36 hours the single cell has become two. Two days later the fertilized egg may have divided twice more to form a microscopic ball of eight cells. In this condition, three and a half days after contact with the sperm, the egg completes its passage through the fallopian tube and enters the uterus.

It is these cells resulting from the early divisions that have become the focus of the stem cell debate. They are pluripotential. This means that they can differentiate into any cell type ultimately found in the human body. You don't have to be a developmental biologist to figure that out. This little cluster of stem cells will eventually differentiate to form the 2000 different cell types in the body and the 100 trillion cells of an adult human: nose, ears, bones, pancreas, liver, brain, spinal cord, and everything else. Until 10 or 20 years ago, embryology students were taught that this was one of biology's great mysteries. Now embryologists are eagerly exploring how to control this differentiation so that pluripotential stem cells can be guided to form brain, liver, pancreas, or anything else that can be helpful in treating human disease and alleviate suffering.

For most opponents to the use of human blastocyst or embryonic stem cells, the issue is straightforward. For them, once egg and sperm nuclei meet and fuse to form a new genome that will be carried by each of the two daughter cells of the first division and then on to all the cells that will ultimate form an embryo, fetus, and baby, you are dealing with a new person. But there are other approaches to obtaining pluripotential stem cells. They can be derived from blastocysts created from in vitro fertilization (sperm meets egg in a test tube or petri dish). Such blastocysts have never seen the inside of a uterus, and by definition, have never formed an embryo.

What if we can form human embryonic stem cells without fertilization? Would the use of these stem cells for research and medical advances violate the sanctity of human life? This can be done, and in fact it is nature's way of reproduction for many species. It is called parthenogenesis—the stimulation of an egg to develop without the introduction of a sperm. It can be achieved by electrical, chemical, or mechanical stimulation. Mammalian nonfertilized eggs have been carried through many stages of development following parthenogenic stimulation. Carrying parthenogenic development through the early rounds of cell division is a no-brainer. These stem cells might have half the number of chromosomes of ordinary stem cells, but we have good scientific evidence to suggest that they can, nevertheless, differentiate into all the cell types of the body. In mammals both the maternal and paternal genomes may be required for embryo development, but an occasional egg will start to develop with two copies of the maternal gene. These usually die early but not until long after they are been through the blastocyst stage, when pluripotential stem cells are present. As stem cells used for therapy in human disease, their genetic constitution would be irrelevant to inheritance because they would not be passed on to succeeding generations. It surprises me that more attention has not been given to parthenogenic activation of eggs for stem cell research, although the first scientific reports are now appearing, particularly from Japanese investigators and subsequently by a small company in Massachusetts that received an inordinate amount of publicity for what seemed like a failed experiment.

The first year I taught embryology at the University of Iowa, it was spring semester and after final exams I left for my summer research at the Marine Biological Laboratory in Woods Hole. There, I received a letter from an anxious young woman in Iowa who had taken the course. She needed some help, it seemed, with a sticky situation at home. Her letter read, "Dear Dr. Segal, Would you please write a letter to my mother immediately, explaining to her about parthenogenesis."

I have emphasized the complexity of the fertilization process and some of the ambiguities of early development to illustrate the difficulty in defining a particular instance when the egg is fertilized, the point in time that some believe defines the origin of new life. This is a debate that has no biological arbiter. The concepts of a new life or "ensoulment" are religious, not biological.

The egg is living before it makes contact with the sperm, and it has the potential even then for leading to a new individual. Moreover, after development begins, it retains a pluripotentiality that complicates the concept of a new life being created at a particular moment. After the first few mitotic divisions of early development, each daughter cell retains the full capability of developing into a complete embryo and proceeding through normal development, so that a single fertilization can lead to many individuals. With modern techniques of assisted reproduction, each of the fully potential daughter cells could be held in a frozen state for many years before being re-implanted and carried through a full pregnancy and normal development. This means that genetically identical twins or triplets could be raised each a few years older than the others. The practitioners of assisted reproduction, as far as we know, have not yet achieved this example of what may be feasible. Freezing and thawing unfertilized eggs is routine; freezing and thawing fertilized eggs or dividing eggs is proving to be more difficult. But the experts have served up other manipulations that overcome many of the problems interfering with fertility. For example, adding cytoplasm from a younger woman's egg can recondition an older woman's egg. After in vitro fertilization, the improved egg can be transferred to the uterus of a third woman.

Now the story of starting a new life begins to get a little complicated. A sperm from either a husband or a donor meets or is injected into an egg with chromosomes of one woman and cytoplasm of another woman, and after nine months, a third woman delivers a baby. Welcome the baby with three mothers: chromosomal mother, cytoplasmic mother, and gestational mother. That calculates out to be at least 12 ways to make a baby, in addition to the old-fashioned way.

My comments are not intended to criticize the field of assisted reproduction, now a major industry. Let me differentiate between the remarkable and praiseworthy success that has brought great joy to thousands of couples who thought they would not be able to have children of their own, and the adventurous undertakings of a few in the field who fail to keep ethical considerations in the forefront of their efforts in assisted reproduction. I served on a Presidential Commission on Population in Washington, D.C., and was assigned the task of reviewing advances in the biology of human reproduction. Cloning had become a familiar term by then, although it would be many years before we learned about Dolly the sheep. My prognosis was that cloning would happen in animals and that human cloning would probably be attempted by a group consisting of "a wealthy sponsor, an ambitious gynecologist, and a publicity-seeking laboratory scientist, using cells from one of the above." We know enough about the scientific limitations in animal cloning to know that in the process of creating one apparently successful clone, there will be a multitude of dead, dying, or deformed clones. I do not believe in legislating restrictions on science, and certainly disapprove of regulatory edicts with political motivation, but I believe that in this field science must hold itself to ethical standards that are beyond reproach.

No one speaks monolithically for science, so that the voices of many fringe groups or individuals are frequently heard on the cloning issue.

The leader of one group, who actually claims that we are all clones of ancient ancestors, is taken seriously enough to be given a seat at congressional hearings. It makes me wonder whether the committee staffers who scheduled the hearings were more interested in garnering facts or publicity. Tom Murray, the president of the Hastings Center, the respected bioethics research center in Garrison, New York, was also at those hearings and wrote eloquently about the realities and ethics of cloning: "You do not need to be a professional bioethicist to see that trying to make a child by cloning, at this stage in the technology, would be a gross violation of international standards protecting people from overreaching scientists, a blatant example of immoral human experimentation." I am in total agreement.

Returning to the normal progression of development, four days after fertilization the egg is a cluster of about 100 cells, which are beginning to divide more rapidly. This stage corresponds to about day 19 or 20 of the menstrual cycle, roughly a week before the next expected menses. The cluster of cells remains unattached for one or two days and assumes the shape of a signet ring: an inner mass of cells encircled by a single row of nourishing cells. The inner cell mass will become the embryo, and the surrounding layer of cells will be the embryo's contribution to the placenta. The fertilized egg gets right to work in differentiating these cells from the embryo proper because this is how it is going to become attached to the mother in order to receive nutrition. This pre-embryo state is called the blastocyst. Little development occurs while the blastocyst remains free in the uterus. It measures about 3 millimeters in diameter (about the size of this letter o) and may float unattached for one or two days. Under the proper conditions the outer ring of cells nestles into the endometrium on the fifth or sixth day and begins to form the placenta. The inner cell mass, after several more days of cell divisions and internal rearrangements, becomes a human embryo. Once in the uterus, about five days after the fertilization process started, the blastocyst needs to attach to the uterine wall to obtain nourishment for further development. It has used up all the nutrients stored in the egg.

While the egg's maturation has been taking place, an integrated sequence is also occurring to ensure a protective and supportive nesting place in the uterus. During the first half of the menstrual cycle, before ovulation, the ovary secretes estrogen in ever-increasing amounts. This stimulates the lining of the uterus (the endometrium) to proliferate and to increase its blood supply. The final surge of estrogen production heralds (and also induces) a mid-cycle peak in the LH level. Ovulation follows within 24 hours, and at about this time ovarian steroid production switches to predominantly progesterone. In response, the cells of the endometrium become still bigger and more numerous. The endometrial glands grow rapidly in length and thickness and begin to accumulate fluid. The entire endometrial surface, by the 20th day of the cycle, has become a highly vascular, spongy nest ready to accept, protect, and nurture a fertilized and dividing egg, should one arrive from the fallopian tube. Once it settles in this supportive nesting place, by definition, the signet-ring–shaped blastocyst becomes an embryo.

At this point, the uterus is under the influence of progesterone. In a nonfertile month, the ovary, failing to receive hormonal signals in the blood indicating that there is a developing blastocyst present, starts to shut down progesterone production about 10 days after ovulation. Some four or five days later the level is too low to support the thick uterine lining, so it is sloughed off, and menstruation occurs. If an egg is fertilized, the next expected menstruation must be avoided. For the pregnancy to survive there must be a source of progesterone to continue to support the endometrium. Without it the blastocyst or embryo would pass out with the sloughed-off endometrium and menstrual blood. To prevent this, there must be physiological recognition of pregnancy within the mother.

The uninterrupted presence of progesterone is absolutely essential for the establishment and maintenance of a human pregnancy. Because of its many vital roles in the physiology of human reproduction, it is no exaggeration to assert that with our present system of reproduction, there could be no human life without progesterone. Progesterone prepares the uterine lining for the implantation of a fertilized egg; development of the vascular bed that becomes the maternal part of the placenta requires progesterone. As long as progesterone levels remain elevated, a pregnancy is not interrupted by a subsequent ovulation, and the next expected menstrual flow, which would be disastrous for a fertilized and dividing egg, is averted. Moreover, progesterone prevents uterine contractions that would dislodge a developing embryo or fetus at any stage of pregnancy. All of these are critical roles without which human reproduction, as we know it, could not take place and the species could not survive.

A French scientist and pioneer reproductive endocrinologist, Robert

Courrier, recognized this as early as 1937, shortly after progesterone was discovered. He wrote, "Progesterone is the hormone of the mother, it is indispensable for reproduction." I knew Courrier in his later years after World War II, when he was president of the French National Academy of Science. He had studied the proceedings of the Nazi doctor trials at Nuremberg and learned that German gynecologist C. Clauberg, well known for his early research on progesterone, had participated in reprehensible experiments on human victims. At the trials, documents were presented to prove that the Nazi gynecologist had boasted in a letter to Heinrich Himmler that he had developed at Auschwitz a method by which he could sterilize 1000 women a day. Courrier was determined to make public these atrocities so that the villain's name would carry the disgrace it deserved rather than be remembered in medical history for his contributions to progesterone research. Over the years, I have attempted to continue Courrier's efforts. My colleagues have grown to expect my hand to shoot up at scientific meetings if the Nazi doctor's name is mentioned in connection with a particular test for progesterone—the Clauberg test. I point out that a British biologist, M. K. MacPhail, had published the same information at about the same time and his independent work would be a more respectable reference to use.

Progesterone was named in the early 1930s by George Corner, a professor of anatomy at the University of Rochester. Its name is derived from its function—*pro*tects *gest*ation—and its chemical structure. Corner later became editor-in-chief of the *Transactions of the American Philosophical Society* in Philadelphia. He also spent some of his post-retirement years in New York City, writing the history of the Rockefeller Institute for Medical Research. Always a modest man, Corner credited colleagues who preceded him and his contemporary co-workers for various parts of the discovery, but his was the seminal work that proved that progesterone exists, that it is produced in the ovary, and that without it there can be no pregnancy.

When I first arrived on the Rockefeller Institute (later Rockefeller University) campus, the laboratory that was being outfitted for me was not yet completed. Corner graciously allowed me to use his laboratory so that I could continue my research. It was there that I became acquainted with some of his younger associates with whom I formed lifelong friendships, including Elsimar Coutinho of Brazil, who later became an important contributor to contraceptive research, and Tapani

Luukkainen of Finland, another major figure in the field of contraception. Coutinho discovered the injectable contraceptives that became DepoProvera and Lunelle, and Luukkainen was the main developer of the intrauterine system Mirenar. Each of these contraceptives uses a derivative of progesterone which is not surprising, considering the laboratory in which Coutinho and Luukkainen received their training in the endocrinology of reproduction.

The synchrony of maturation, release, and fertilization of the egg, on the one hand, and preparation of the uterus as a proper environment for implantation, on the other, is achieved because the hormones involved in each process have such exquisitely integrated and interrelated functions. Consider the implications of the hormonal events of a typical cycle. After ovulation the gonadal steroid hormones enter the bloodstream and, as their levels increase, serve as a signal to the pituitary to shut down secretion of LH and FSH. The progressive decline in the concentration of the pituitary gonadotropins in the blood prevents any supplementary ovulations that would interfere in the event that fertilization had occurred. Once it is clear that a cycle has been infertile, there is an immediate signal to the brain to initiate the events that prepare for an egg release the next month. The brain recognizes the decline in blood steroid concentrations late in the cycle, and this prompts a rise in LH and FSH. Although menstruation intervenes, signaling the end of the previous cycle, the new cycle has already begun in response to the secretion of LH and FSH. Follicular maturation proceeds, and with it the development of a new egg and a new wave of steroid hormone production. At about mid-cycle, rising estrogen levels trigger the preovulatory surge of LH, and ovulation results.

My friend James Bradbury used to teach reproductive endocrinology to medical students at the University of Iowa. He gave a brilliant lecture in which he compared this system to the thermostatic control of heating a house, automatically turning on and off in response to need. Fundamentally, it does work like a thermostat, turning the pituitary's production of gonadotropins on and off in response to the blood hormone levels as perceived by a specialized region of the brain.

The human reproductive system did not evolve to be fruitless. If fertilization takes place in a given month, physiological recognition of pregnancy becomes essential. First, the forthcoming menstruation must be avoided. An uninterrupted supply of progesterone is needed to maintain the uterine wall. It cannot start to break down as it may have done every previous month of the woman's reproductive years. To achieve this, the blastocyst sends out a molecular message alerting the ovary to its presence. Even before the early blastocyst implants in the uterine wall, its outer cells copiously produce a gonadotropin-like molecule called human chorionic gonadotropin (hCG). It is very similar in structure and function to pituitary LH and is the famous hormone of pregnancy. It is the chemical molecule that virtually all pregnancy tests are designed to identify. When the most sensitive tests are used, hCG can be found in a woman's blood or urine at least a week before the first day of the next expected period. By producing hCG, the blastocyst is beginning to take responsibility for its own fate. Human chorionic gonadotropin stimulates the corpus luteum to maintain the production of progesterone beyond the time of the first expected menstrual period.

The first weeks after fertilization are hazardous for the new conceptus. About one-third of all fertilized eggs are lost in these early weeks, most without the woman ever being aware of conceiving. We now know from cytogenetic studies of recovered samples that many of the lost blastocysts carry lethal mutations or vital gene deficiencies that determine this fate.

A second critical period lies ahead. The corpus luteum, in spite of maximal stimulation by hCG, has a limited life span. Before this time limit is reached, at about the eighth week of gestation, a new solution has to be found to maintain the flow of progesterone. By then the life-supporting placenta has formed with both a maternal and a fetal component. The closely juxtaposed maternal and fetal blood supplies enable maternal nutrients to be passed to the fetus. As the life span of the corpus luteum draws to an end, the placenta begins to produce sufficient quantities of progesterone to maintain the pregnancy. To pass the first crisis, in other words, the embryo produces a gonadotropin that stimulates maternal hormone production. To meet the second crisis, the developing embryo assumes the required endocrine function, thus becoming self-sufficient in this respect. By the eighth or ninth week, the pregnancy can continue even if the maternal ovaries cease to function or are removed.

This period of transition from maternal to placental progesterone production is another vulnerable point in pregnancy associated with a high incidence of miscarriages. More and more throughout pregnancy, the fetus and its placenta take charge of the pregnancy's hormonal requirements until the fetal–placental unit produces the hormones and enzymes that will facilitate delivery, even preparing for the newborn's first meal by producing the hormones that stimulate development of the mother's mammary glands and start milk production.

Other vertebrate species base survival not on nurturing and protecting an individual offspring, but on the production of huge numbers of eggs with the expectation that some will survive to reach sexual maturity and reproduce. Human evolution has created a system to produce a single offspring, nurtured and protected in the woman's uterus, nursed and cared for after birth. The result is a method of reproducing that is physiologically efficient for the individual and effective to assure continuity of the species. This pattern of reproduction has provided enough flexibility for survival from nomadic existence throughout all the changing circumstances of human history.

In the evolutionary development of animals that deliver a single living offspring instead of multiple numbers of eggs to be developed outside of the mother, the reproductive adaptations from the more primitive strategy to the nurtured-offspring approach have occurred mainly in the female. These adaptations have built into the system reproduction efficiency, elimination of large-scale reproductive wastage, and maximal chances of survival for an individual newborn. I mentioned earlier that the multiplication phase of ooctyes is restricted to fetal life. This is extremely important and was a necessary change from the more primitive systems in which the ovaries are simple egg sacs that can fill the female's entire abdomen during breeding season. Along with this, the development of a sophisticated follicle system that provides each potential egg with its own chamber within the ovary was an essential anatomical adaptation. The ovarian follicle includes the egg, supportive nurse cells, and cells capable of producing either estrogen or progesterone. This gets all the machinery in place for what will be needed for the hormonal cycle of a woman.

The ovarian follicle was recognized early in the study of human anatomy but, in those days before the microscope, its purpose was misread. In 1672 when the Dutch anatomist Regner de Graff described the fluid-filled ovarian chambers, he thought they were the eggs. The label Graffian follicle still remains in medical usage. Nearly 200 years after de Graff, the accurate relationship between the follicle of the ovary and the egg became clear when Karl von Baer visualized the tiny human egg inside the follicle. Later, the light microscope and the electron microscope revealed even greater complexity of the ovary and the key role it plays in the menstrual cycle of the human female.

Adaptations were not confined to the ovary. The female genome coalesced all the genetic mechanisms required for the sequence of events from individual ovum maturation through gestation, delivery, and nurturing, paying attention to even obscure but essential details like the timely production of a hormone to relax the ligaments of the woman's pelvis during delivery so that the baby's head can slip through.

The male reproductive process does not share evidence of the sophisticated evolutionary adaptations found in the female. The male's hormonal system is not cyclical, and the multiplication phase of primordial germ cells (the primitive stem cells that will give rise to sperm) in the testis is not restricted. The structure of the human testis might be characterized as generic. A microscopist looking at a human testis sees a structure remarkably similar to that of a frog, fish, or mouse— a compact body of tightly convoluted tubules held intact by a shiny, fibrous sheath. The seminiferous tubules of the human testis, in which sperm production takes place, would extend for several miles if straightened out.

The human male produces countless spermatozoa in a lifetime, a trait reminiscent of lower vertebrate species that derive survival value from the copious release of sperm in the general vicinity of unfertilized eggs discharged by the female into sea water, tidal marshes, or ponds. The man's billions of sperm come from the 1000–2000 primitive germ cells that migrate into the embryonic testis before the end of the second month of intrauterine life. The massive number of sperm that will ultimately be produced is made possible by the way the original cells (called spermatogonia) multiply and because they never stop multiplying. When primary spermatogonia divide, many of the daughter cells are kept in reserve, while others undergo further cell divisions and then complete sperm formation. In contrast to the multiplication phase in the ovary, which is confined to a few months of fetal life, the multiplication phase in the testis begins in the fetal period and continues throughout life. Because there is no significant depletion of germ-cell stores, there is no gradual loss of gamete-producing function as there is in the ovary. The testis goes on producing millions upon millions of spermatozoa, and there always remain additional germ cells with the capability of producing millions more. Although the process of atresia depletes all of the ovary's follicles, thus precipitating menopause, the testis has no such mechanism to end the potential of its reproductive performance. It is not uncommon, however, for the vascular changes of aging to affect the testis or pituitary and indirectly cause a loss of testicular function. There can be, therefore, a "male menopause," or "andropause," but its cause is quite different from the causes of female menopause.

I once did a study on the effect of aging on the human testis and found that about half of octogenarians who were patients in the urology ward had testosterone levels almost the same as young, virile men. When I reported this at grand rounds, the nurses who had helped by collecting urine samples for the hormone assays scolded me for wasting their time and my own. They said they could attest to the sustained libido of these elderly men.

In the course of sperm formation, the two important objectives are the reduction of the chromosome number from the diploid number (46) to the haploid number (23) and the preparation of the sperm for its role in fertilization. A complex series of transformations involving both the cytoplasm and the nucleus changes the large, round immature cells into the elongated and motile sperm. This occurs within the tubules of the testis. The entire cycle from primordial spermatogonia to sperm takes approximately 74 days. It is a process that goes on continuously throughout the miles-long, coiled seminiferous tubules.

The testis, like the ovary, must be stimulated by pituitary gonadotropins to produce sex hormones and sperm. The role of LH is primarily to stimulate the hormone-producing cells that produce testosterone. Testosterone, in turn, has an important effect on the process of sperm production because a high local concentration of the hormone is needed to maintain sperm formation. Follicle-stimulating hormone binds specifically to the cells that nurture developing sperm cells. This implies that its role is in the maintenance of the sperm-developing process, an interpretation supported by the fact that whenever something interferes with sperm production, the level of FSH in circulation tends to rise, suggesting that FSH is not being utilized normally.

The sperm's voyage can be described even though many of its control mechanisms are incompletely understood. A limited number of collecting ducts funnel the spermatozoa coming from the testicular tubules to the epididymis, a long tube convoluted into a compact body adjacent to the testis. These immature sperm are not yet able to fertilize an egg or even to move under their own power. As they pass from the head of the epididymis through its slender body to its distended tail, they become motile, but the final critical changes that enable sperm to fertilize an egg are finally achieved when they reach the female reproductive tract.

From the tail of the epididymis the sperm proceed into the vas deferens, which empties into the urethra below the bladder. Some of the sperm die and are disposed of by white blood cells; others enter the urethra in a steady stream and are carried away in the urine. Vast numbers leave the male tract at ejaculation, when the sperm are forced into the urethra by muscular contractions. These sperm are mixed with the fluid secretions of several accessory glands, including the prostate and seminal vesicles, whose ducts lead into the terminal portion of the vas deferens or into the urethra. Together these elements constitute the semen, which serves primarily as a vehicle to carry the sperm to the vagina. Most of the sperm go no farther. Of the hundreds of millions that are ejaculated, only tens of thousands reach the cervix, which is the entry to the uterus. Here there is a further attrition, so that only a few thousand reach the uterus proper. A few hundred spermatozoa ultimately complete the journey to the upper part of the fallopian tube, where one of them may fertilize an egg.

In addition to providing more insight into human biology in general and improved diagnosis and treatment of various diseases and abnormal conditions, increased understanding of the reproductive process can have a direct impact on the human condition. The physician's ability to help people have the children they want through assisted reproduction procedures has increased tremendously. At the same time, contraceptive technology has improved to the point where couples throughout the world can find it easier to reduce their fertility. With advances in contraception, women or couples at any level of motivation can be offered more effective, acceptable, and safe methods that they can voluntarily choose to use.

Reproductive freedom means the ability to have children or to choose not to have children. Science has made major advances to help couples fulfill each of these goals. In the process of these discoveries, science has also achieved phenomenal advances in our understanding of how the hormones of reproduction affect our lives in many other ways. They influence our body structure, blood chemistry, and behavior. They can prevent, cause, or exacerbate illnesses, including cancer. In females, the changing flow of natural hormones controls the transition from prepuberty to adolescence, the reproductive years, and the menopause.

3

The Changing Modern Woman

In a *Peanuts* cartoon Lucy asks Charlie Brown, "Do you think people really change?" He says, "Sure, I feel I've changed a lot this past year." To this Lucy responds, "I meant for the better!"

Women are changing for the better! Nowhere can society claim that women have achieved equity with men, but in many countries they are gaining a more equal role, greater opportunity to fulfill their hopes and aspirations, and autonomy in decisions concerning their own fertility.

The worldwide decline in total fertility rate (TFR), the number of children a woman has in her lifetime, is based on an average calculated country-by-country, but the real significance of the decline is how it affects the individual woman. Does having fewer children make a difference in her personal life, her family life, or in her community role? Does it make a difference to her biologically?

Throughout the world, women have fewer children as they become more educated, receive better health care, enter the workforce, marry at a later age, or participate in community affairs outside of the home. These are some of the social correlates of a decreasing total fertility rate. Analyzing what effect this demographic statistic has on a woman's reproductive life reveals some inescapable biological correlates. Obviously, it reduces her risk of pregnancy-related death or disability. In addition, the lifetime pattern of her reproductive processes changes as the total fertility rate falls. The reproductive biology of modern woman is changing.

Italy has one of the world's lowest total fertility rates. The country's TFR of 1.1 means that Italian women average slightly more than one full-term pregnancy during their reproductive years. Since abortion is not very popular in Catholic Italy, how do they stop from having more pregnancies? There are only two other options: abstinence, including delay in the age of marriage, and contraception, including surgical sterilization. I don't think of Italy as a particularly abstemious society, but the Italians are very efficient users of contraception. In 1979, the last time a survey was done, contraception was used by about 80% of married women. Contraceptive use now is probably even more extensive since the TFR has declined to its present level since the time of that survey.

We also have information on what contraceptives Italian women used at that time. Fourteen percent were using the pill, which usually inhibits ovulation. The rest were using methods that do not inhibit ovulation. Accounting for the 3% of women of childbearing age who are pregnant or breast-feeding in any given year, and some who are infertile, this means that roughly 80% of Italian women in the reproductive years were having regular menstrual cycles in 1979. The percentage has probably gone up a few percentage points because more Italian women are using contraceptive methods that do not inhibit ovulation. Use of IUDs has gained at the expense of oral contraceptives, and the condom has returned to favor with rising concern about sexually transmitted diseases, including HIV/AIDS. The influx of immigrants from Eastern Europe and North Africa may have changed the statistics somewhat, but not the overall picture.

This means that most Italian women are ovulating and menstruating regularly from menarche at age 12 to menopause at age 48, except for a short time to have their one baby and a few months of breast-feeding—about 15–18 months altogether. The rest of that 36-year stretch of their adolescent and adult life, Italian women are having menstrual cycle after menstrual cycle, year in and year out, even though they have no intention of getting pregnant. Yet, making it possible to get pregnant is what the cycle is all about! The total number of periods will be 400–480, depending on the exact ages of the menarche and menopause and the influence on ovulation of factors like stress or vigorous exercise.

In all of Europe, where 35 countries are at or below replacement level of fertility, the pattern is pretty much the same as the Italian model. In countries that have reached but not fallen below replacement level, with a TFR around 2, the same pattern of many years of menstrual cycles prevails, with two time-outs instead of one. This prevails in the United States, Canada, Australia, New Zealand, and 10 Asian countries including Japan, China, South Korea, and Taiwan. Moreover, regular menstrual cycles are becoming characteristic for women in traditionally high-fertility countries where pregnancy or nursing customarily occupied most of their reproductive years. As the TFR continues to decline and the duration of breast-feeding shortens around the world, the number of women who spend most of their reproductive years ovulating and menstruating will grow. Countries with fertility near or below replacement level already account for just less than half the world's total population. For about half the world's population, in other words, women in their reproductive years will have one or two pregnancies and for the rest of their reproductive years they will be menstruating regularly. Fading is the image of poor women in poor countries, clasping a nursing baby, carrying another on their back, holding a toddler's hand, and pregnant.

Does this mean that having regular ovulatory cycles and periods is natural? Not if you consider the biological norm natural. I first started thinking about this when I was doing studies in India on the biology of reproduction of the rhesus monkey. These primates have ovulatory and menstrual cycles similar to those of humans. I couldn't understand why none of the animals brought into the laboratory from their natural habitat, whether from rural areas or urban parks, was a mature, menstruating female, so I accompanied the animal handlers on a collecting trip to find out. (At that time, incidentally, the rural collecting area was out near New Delhi's international airport. Now urban spread has expanded the city well beyond the airport and pushed the troops of monkeys farther and farther away from their original territory.) I was pleased to see the gentleness of the collecting operation as one would expect in nonviolent India, where Hindus adore Hanuman, the monkey god, but it soon became evident to me that in the wild, there were no nonpregnant mature females! All were either pregnant, lactating, or both. This was the biological norm and what was natural for these primates. The menstruation we observed in our laboratory colonies was an artifact of the unnatural circumstances of their environment with males and females separated.

Since the dawn of the human epoch and over the long sweep of human history, it is likely that ovulation has been infrequent and episodic. In constant contact with men, it would have been extraordinary for a woman to ovulate and menstruate regularly. Like the nonhuman primates I observed, ovulation and menstruation were naturally suppressed as a result of pregnancies followed by long periods of breast-feeding. That was the reproductive system that evolved under the control of the human genome.

From the time of the menarche, perhaps even before the first menstruation, early woman became pregnant and thereafter was either pregnant or lactating continuously during her short life span. Only when the infant began to receive supplementary nourishment and breast-feeding diminished would occasional ovulations resume. In that era of high maternal death rates, there were undoubtedly motherless infants who needed to be cared for by other lactating women, so that surrogate nursing would also have contributed to suppressing ovulatory cycles.

A woman would often become re-impregnated without an intervening menstruation. A new pregnancy and period of lactation would follow, extending the amenorrhea. Even today, in any given month in countries with high fertility and prolonged lactation, there are probably more women of reproductive age not menstruating than there are menstruating.

Modern woman has essentially the same genetic constitution as her ancestral sisters. Yet, her reproductive pattern has changed from the era of incessant reproduction to the era of incessant menstruation. Throughout most of the historical presence of women on earth, regular periods have not been the pattern of their reproductive years. The change began when fertility and breast-feeding started to decline in the 1800s around the time of the industrial revolution. Colonial women in America, for example, had an average of eight children in their lifetime. That many full-term pregnancies with the subsequent periods of breast-feeding and the inevitable miscarriages left little calendar time during a woman's reproductive years for regular periods.

For early humans, the mortality of females beyond puberty must have been much higher than that of men due principally to reproductive causes. Estimated life expectancy was 33 years for males and 28 years for females. Women reached puberty late, generally after 18 years of age. The supposition that early *Homo sapiens* woman would have spent most of her adult life pregnant or breast-feeding until an early death is reinforced by anthropologic evidence indicating that the number of surviving adult males exceeded females by the proportion of three to one. Death of females must have been caused primarily by the complications of pregnancy and childbirth.

Because child mortality was also high, the population did not grow to any great extent, despite these repeated pregnancies. Even today in countries where health services are severely inadequate 1 of 5 children does not reach its fifth birthday, and 1 in 20 women dies of a pregnancy-related cause. The genetically endowed extra survivability of females compared to males would not have spared Paleolithic women from the hazards of pregnancy, childbirth, and postpartum health risks. The unfavorable circumstances under which women live even in some twenty-first-century countries are sufficiently deplorable to override this genetic advantage, so that death rates for women exceeds those of men. In Uganda and Nepal, life expectancy of women is actually lower than that of men, a highly unusual, counter-biological statistic.

Some primitive cultures in today's world maintain the reproductive behavior of their predecessors from the preagricultural past. Child-bearing begins with sexual maturation. The women experience, as their ancestors did, alternating periods of gestation with breast-feeding on demand, throughout all their fertile years. Anthropologists find striking differences compared to modern women in the reproductive patterns of these hunter–gatherer societies, believed to be unchanged from the patterns of 100,000 years ago. With an average of six pregnancies and nearly three years of breast-feeding per child, !Kung San women of southern Africa or tribes in Australia are pregnant or lactating for nearly 25 years of their lives and experience only 50 to 150 menstrual periods in a lifetime. At either extreme of this range the number is far lower than the 400-plus of women in more advanced societies. But even this reduced number of menstrual cycles is probably greater than the number experienced by gatherer women in prehistoric times when the age of menarche was older and life expectancy was shorter because life carried greater risks, survival was has harder, and food was more difficult to come by than for today's surviving tribes.

From an evolutionary point of view, the human system of reproduction and nurturing, with its single, highly dependent offspring and
its checks and balances, has survival value for the species. It requires
that infant care is programmed into the human makeup and that the
infant will receive adequate attention to get started in life before another one is born. From the individual's perspective, it means that maternal instinct had to be programmed into the genetic control of the
human reproductive process.

Humans have an inherited propensity for nurturing behavior. The
hormones of pregnancy prime an expectant mother for maternal behavior, but genetic influences that lie much further back in both women
and men's life history constantly evoke a nurturing instinct. For the
human reproductive system to be successful, this instinct needs to be
strong enough to assure that most women will want to bear at least
one child, despite the costs and sacrifices of so doing. (This implies that
my example country, Italy, with a TFR of 1.1, has already reached its
limit to low fertility because the strong biological predisposition to
have children will ultimately override the environmental factors that
are influencing fertility decision making.)

The human genome established an era of incessant reproduction that
served the species well. How else can you view moving from the origin
of the species to a global population of 6 billion? But modern woman
with essentially the same genetic endowment now has a totally different
pattern of reproduction. Environmental influences have taken over, and
the reproductive system has been able to adapt. Without genetic
change, we have moved from the hundreds of thousands of years of
maximal childbearing to the relatively recent era of an occasional pregnancy and many years of continuous fruitless ovulation and menstruation during a woman's reproductive life span. The genes that influence
reproductive performance can accommodate this large a shift.

Not all reproductive systems found in nature are that flexible. Some
birds are programmed to brood five eggs a season, for example. If you
take one egg out of the nest, the female will lay another, if you remove
two eggs, she'll replace them with two more. If you surreptitiously
sneak in smooth, round stones, she'll believe that her brood is full and
hold back the corresponding number of eggs. It's the old shell game!

The obstetrical toad of West Africa is another example of nature's
potential for inflexibility. The female is programmed to lay her eggs at
a certain fixed time in the early spring, timed to correspond with the

expected presence of ample ponds and puddles from spring rains. She will lay her eggs at that time, come rain or shine. If the rains are late, however, there is no standing water to harbor the fertilized eggs while they develop into tadpoles. There is no built-in system for changing the timetable; the females lay their eggs anyway. All would be lost except for an ingenious fail-safe mechanism. The males are genetically programmed to carry the jelly-coated egg clutches on their back, covering them with a protective cover of mucus until the rains fall and the eggs can be safely deposited in the needed water.

I had heard about this admirable amphibian from my friend, the late Professor Louis Gallien of the Sorbonne, who had traveled to Africa to study the endocrinology of the obstetrical toad's reproductive process. In recent years, one theory to explain the mysterious decline and disappearance of many amphibian species around the world has been hormonal disruption caused by unknown environmental factors. I was saddened to read lately that Gallien's obstetrical toads, inhabitants of earth since before the emergence of *Homo sapiens*, are on the endangered list.

In contrast, the adaptability of the human system without genomic shifts is extraordinary, but this carries with it changes in nonreproductive functions as well. The introduction of almost 35 years of ovulatory cycles, including monthly menstruations, changes the woman's body in ways that have both short-term and long-term health-related implications. The short-term problems are known to most women: the monthly pain of menstrual cramps, living with the symptoms of premenstrual syndrome, onset of migraines, endometriosis, and for millions of women around the world, the lethargy and tiredness caused by iron-deficiency anemia.

Menstrual pain (dysmenorrhea) is caused by cramping of the smooth muscles of the uterus. It can be so severe that a woman cannot carry out her daily activities at home or at work. The condition occurs among such a large percentage of women that it is the most common cause for visits to gynecologists. Someone who suffers the monthly anguish of dysmenorrhea does not have to be convinced that it is a serious woman's health problem. Apart from palliative relief obtained by using painkillers, the only way to overcome the problem is to prevent menstruation. This is because in the normal course of the hormonal changes of a menstrual cycle, the production of prostaglandin is inevitable at the end of the menstrual month, and this internal hormone has a strong effect in causing the contraction and cramping of the uterine muscle. That's why prostaglandin inhibitors like aspirin or ibuprofen can help.

Endometriosis is another common cause of pelvic pain in women of reproductive age. It was probably rare before the era of regular menstruation because it is both caused by and regularly exacerbated by the menstrual period. Endometriosis is a painful condition in which cells from the uterine lining grow outside the uterus, in the pelvic cavity. Most doctors agree that it is a result of the backflow of menstrual blood through the fallopian tube during menstruation. Instead of all the blood lost from the broken blood vessels in the uterine lining during a menstruation passing out through the vagina, about half flows into the pelvic cavity, where the hemoglobin is broken down and the iron resorbed. This normal process serves to conserve iron stores. Sometimes this retrograde flow carries with it cells or fragments of the uterine lining that attach onto other organs and tissues in the abdominal or pelvic cavity. They usually come to rest on areas of inflammation as, for example, the point at which the ovary has a ruptured follicle at its surface. Each month, these fragments respond to the woman's hormonal changes the same way that the uterine lining does. This can mean growing eight to ten times their original size. Depending on where the fragments are located, they can cause extreme pain both during the normal course of the cycle (dysmenorrhea) and especially during intercourse (dyspareunia).

Women who have access to good health care facilities can get relief, usually by surgery, certain hormone treatments, or with pain-killing medications. Without adequate medical care, attacks of endometriosis pain can be a monthly torment for women. Not infrequently, it becomes the reason for the extreme surgical treatment, an elective hysterectomy with removal of the ovaries.

Once considered a disease of the well-educated and affluent who tend to delay the age of first childbirth, endometriosis is becoming more common around the world as women marry later and reduce the frequency of pregnancies. The World Health Organization considers endometriosis the major cause of women's infertility and estimates that it afflicts about 10% of the world's women of reproductive age. This means that about 150 million women suffer from endometriosis, whether or not it has been diagnosed. Often the monthly suffering is simply considered "women's problems," and the condition is left undiagnosed, untreated, and unrelieved.

With declining fertility around the world, the numbers are bound to grow, and suffering from endometriosis will worsen unless simple remedies can be found that are easy to distribute and administer, even in the absence of an advanced health care delivery system. Surgery is not going to be the solution for most of the world's women who suffer from endometriosis. Suppressing menstruation can both reduce the chances of endometriosis becoming established in the first place and eliminate the monthly hormonal changes that exacerbate the pain and suffering with each menstrual period or with intercourse.

Specialists have learned that certain diseases flare up in women patients at the time of their periods. This category is referred to as catamenial diseases, taking the name from the fact that the diseases occur with menstruation. Neurologists find, for example, that some women with epilepsy have seizures only at the time of their periods. This would be called catamenial epilepsy, and the treatment, using hormones in addition to standard drugs, might be somewhat different from the treatment for other forms of epilepsy. A nurse who specializes in patient-directed management of diabetes told me that her young female patients with type I diabetes have a much more complicated insulin management once they reach puberty and their periods begin. At the end of each menstrual month, they require higher doses of insulin to control their blood sugar levels. This is probably due to progesterone-induced differences in insulin receptors and therefore the potency of insulin when it is taken at different stages of the cycle.

For some women, migraine and asthma attacks can also fall in the category of catamenial conditions. Arthritis sufferers experience more joint pain and stiffness during menstruation. There is even a rare condition called "menstrual arthritis" in which arthritis pain occurs exclusively at the time of the menses. Irritable bowel syndrome is a common, painful disorder that affects women as much as 20 times more frequently than men. The explanation for the gender difference is that it is associated with changing hormone levels during the menstrual cycle. When the menstrual cycle is completely eliminated (by pregnancy or hormone treatment), women experience significant improvement.

Menstruation contributes significantly to iron-deficiency anemia. This decreases the body's supply of oxygen, thereby depressing the capacity to perform physical labor. Iron deficiency also reduces learning performance. The body has very efficient mechanisms for conserving iron, but the blood loss associated with menstruation causes the depletion of iron stores. Because iron is required to form hemoglobin, the oxygen-carrying protein of the red blood cell, iron deficiency can result in anemia or can worsen a preexisting anemic condition caused by malnutrition, parasitic infection, or other causes. Consequently, as the number of menstruations increase, so does the risk of iron deficiency. About 30% of the world's population, mostly women, is anemic. In terms of absolute numbers of individuals, anemia is undoubtedly the disease most affected by menstrual blood loss. For countless millions of malnourished or parasite-infected women around the world already suffering from chronic anemia, the blood loss associated with regular menstruation causes depletion in iron stores that can worsen the condition. For these women, anemia must be recognized as a serious consequence of repetitive menstruations.

I have planned international field trials on new contraceptive methods in which women with a low blood iron level (measured as hemoglobin) would not be included. Requiring a hemoglobin value of 12 (g/dL), considered normal in the United States, meant that almost every woman who wanted to enter the study in countries like India or Bangladesh had to be excluded. In poor countries, the main reasons for this high rate of anemia are malnutrition and parasitic diseases, but these causes do not explain the fact that menstruating women require twice as much iron intake as men to maintain normal iron levels in the blood. To absorb enough iron to make up for the blood loss during menstruation, a woman needs to have in her diet up to 40 milligrams of iron per day. For men, the recommended dietary requirement is half that amount. When women stop menstruating at menopause their anemia lessens.

Iron-deficiency anemia is not only a condition of the poorer countries. In a study done by pediatricians at the Johns Hopkins Children's Center, the blood of 700 Baltimore schoolgirls was tested and revealed that 100 had iron levels below normal, in the range considered to be anemic. High-dose iron supplements for two months raised their iron levels and substantially improved their scores in memorization and verbal learning. Another Baltimore study demonstrated the benefits of using Norplant contraceptives to avoid second pregnancies in teenage mothers. Too bad that study protocol didn't include following the blood iron levels. It might have demonstrated that a secondary benefit for these young mothers was an improvement in blood iron. We do know, however, that women who start using Norplant when their blood iron is low experience an elevation in values during the first year of use, bringing the level back to normal. This is because the amount of menstrual-like blood loss when using Norplant is far less than the blood loss of regular periods.

Even more of a threat than a normal period in causing iron-deficiency anemia is menorrhagia, the medical term that describes excessive blood loss during menstruation. No one understands why it happens that some women have an extraordinarily heavy flow. Menorrhagia is usually defined as a vaginal blood loss of more than 100 milliliters of blood a month. Menorrhagia is believed to affect as many as 20% of women and is another of the menstrual cycle-related health disorders that bring women to their gynecologist's office at a high frequency. The condition can even be life threatening and is sometimes treated surgically by some form of curettage or, in extreme situations, by hysterectomy.

Surveys reveal that up to 90% of American women experience episodic, short-term problems associated with monthly periods. About half experience pain for one or two days of their periods, and about 10% have so much pain that their daily routine is disrupted for one to three days a month. A survey of Swedish women revealed about the same result. Two-thirds of the Swedish women in the study reported that they use painkillers during menstruation both for cramps and migraine headaches. If you ask American or Swedish women about their complaints regarding menstruation, they will emphasize pain, mood changes, and the inconvenience.

My Brazilian colleague Elsimar Coutinho wrote a book in Portuguese on menstruation, which we later joined in transforming into an expanded version for an international audience. Called *Is Menstruation Obsolete?* and published by Oxford University Press, the book attracted a great deal of attention from the media and sent reporters out to get reactions from women to the idea of doing away with periods. A typical response was, "Not having my period is complete freedom. I never have to worry about it coming early and catching me my surprise. Not to mention the serious cramps I always used to experience." This comment illustrates the month-to-month problems women associate with their periods.

Less well-known is that the modern pattern of incessant menstrual cycles is linked to other major long-term health risks for women. There is a correlation between number of cycles and the risk of certain reproductive tract cancers. Ovarian cancer is a much-feared gynecologic cancer; it is very aggressive and frequently fatal. In large epidemiological studies, clear trends of decreasing risk of invasive ovarian cancer were evident with increasing numbers of pregnancies and extended duration of breast-feeding. Suppressing ovulations by taking the pill also reduces the risk of ovarian cancer.

What the three risk-reducing conditions, pregnancy, breast-feeding, and oral contraception, have in common is that they suppress ovulation and menstruation. Breast-feeding adds additional protection with each month continued, up to six months, the time when breakthrough ovulations can be expected. The extent of the protective effect is quite impressive. The first pregnancy reduces the risk about 40%, and with each of the next pregnancies there is a slight added protection. Any period of breast-feeding reduces the risk of ovarian cancer by about 25%, and protection increases with the duration of lactation. Women who use oral contraceptives for at least six months reduce their risk by 40%.

The corollary of this information is that as the number of ovulatory menstrual cycles in a woman's reproductive history increases, the risk of ovarian cancer increases. Women who have never been pregnant have an increased risk. There is a rational explanation of these facts that raises the question whether incessant ovulation is natural. Every time an egg is released at ovulation, there is a slight tear in the surface of the ovary so that the egg can be set free to enter the fallopian tube. That trauma to the ovarian surface has to be repaired by rapidly dividing cells through the process of mitosis. An abundance of dividing cells risks that the proliferation may continue unchecked as a result of an abnormal mitosis. Considering this in connection with the falling fertility rate, it means that for the one egg an Italian woman is going to have fertilized in her reproductive years, she will experience about 450 slight tears in the ovarian wall that will have to be patched up by active mitosis and cell division. The question is whether scientists can chart an increase in the rate of ovarian cancer with decline in fertility. We don't have an answer because there are many confounding factors that make it difficult to establish a direct cause and effect between the disease and a single factor. Although life-threatening, ovarian cancer is not highly prevalent, so it would take huge numbers of cases before an association between ovarian cancer and number of menstrual cycles could be demonstrated epidemiologically.

Cancer of the uterine lining, the endometrium, is also a life-threatening gynecological disease. The relationship of this cancer to number of ovarian cycles is similar to that described for ovarian cancer: the fewer cycles, the greater the protection. The risk of endometrial cancer in women who have used ovulation-inhibiting oral contraceptives for at least two years is about 40% less than among women who have never used the pill. The number of periods a woman has between menarche and menopause also influences the extent of risk: the greater number of cycles, the greater the risk.

These observations also have a biological explanation. Endometrial cancer is an estrogen-induced cancer. A woman's ovaries produce the highest level of estrogen during her cycle just before ovulation. This means that month after month, high estrogen levels without the modulating effect of the second ovarian hormone, progesterone, stimulate the endometrial tissue. As the endometrial cells respond to the stimulatory effect of estrogen, there is considerable mitotic activity, creating the opportunity for unwanted mutations that can start a cancer. It is only after ovulation that the rise in progesterone secretion begins and serves to protect the uterine lining from further exposure to unopposed estrogen.

Breast cancer risk is also linked to cycle frequency, and the present evidence suggests that the fewer menstruations in a woman's lifetime, the lower the risk. Consequently, the longer the period of breast-feeding after each pregnancy, the lower the risk of breast cancer.

Listing the risks of regular ovulatory cycles may be one sided. Could it be that there are overlooked health benefits to the ovarian cycle and menstruation that have nothing to do with pregnancy? Mothers around the globe teach their daughters that "the curse" is necessary to cleanse their insides. If my wife had told that to our preadolescent daughters, they would have asked, "Why don't boys have to have their insides cleaned?" It's a good question and the answer is they don't, and neither do girls or women. Simply put, a human menstrual period is the by-product of a month in which there has been no fertilization. It has no other purpose. It is not necessary to "cleanse" the woman's system or to eliminate toxins.

There have been theories for other roles, but none has taken hold because of the lack of substantiating evidence. One theory proposed that menstruation is a means of getting rid of infectious bacteria that come into the uterus hanging on to the tail of sperm. It is hard to understand the biological benefit of waiting until the end of the month to get rid of bacteria introduced into the uterus days or even weeks earlier. There is also strong contradictory evidence based on studies showing that women have the highest risk of reproductive tract infection during menstruation. This would seem to question the notion that menstruation plays a role as a cleansing or purgative mechanism. Another hypothesis suggests that in evolution, menstruation plays a role in eliminating abnormal embryos. It is true that a large percentage of fertilized human eggs are spontaneously discharged, many at the time of the first menstruation after fertilization. But in this circumstance, the menstrual flow is simply the flushing-out mechanism and not causal in rejecting the genetically impaired product of conception. We know of no mechanism by which the maternal system can determine the genetic quality of a newly forming embryo. In fact, in human pregnancy there is a built-in immunological mechanism to assure that the maternal system does not treat the genetically different embryo as a foreign invader and reject it.

Why women bleed so profusely during menstruation (up to 100 milliliters of blood and its precious iron stores can be lost each month) has never been understood. This copious monthly bleeding is a uniquely human characteristic. An imaginative new theory proposed by Dr. Jennifer Weil suggests that in ancestral times, in spite of its biological cost to women, overt menses had the major advantage of serving as a signal, alerting males to a female's fertility. The time of optimal chances of fertility in women is not easily detectable by behavioral or biological clues as it is in other species. According to this original theory, selective identification of fertile, nonpregnant females would have had an adaptive advantage for the species. It makes very good sense.

When describing total fertility rate, I explained that there is a direct correlation between TFR and the prevalence of contraceptive use. The greater the use of contraceptives in a country, the lower the TFR. There is another correlation with TFR to consider. Along with lower fertility, life expectancy of women increases. Since I started using the examples of Italy and India, let me continue with these countries. Italy in 2000 had a life expectancy at birth for females of 82 years. An infant girl born in India the same year could expect to live to age 64. Just eight years earlier, in Italy the life expectancy of a female was 78 and in India it was 54. This trend toward longer life expectancy will continue, particularly in the world's poorer countries that are not affected by AIDS. It is projected that by 2025 India's female life expectancy will reach 76, and Italy will stabilize at about 84. This means that Italian and Indian women will live for more postmenopausal years. This, too, is part of the legacy of a lower TFR, and it is happening throughout the world.

A woman may spend as much as one-third of her lifetime in the menopausal years. During these years, because of hormonal and other bodily changes, women are subjected to a series of health problems; all are serious, some are life-threatening. During menopause women have an increased risk of cardiovascular disease, including high blood pressure, heart attack, and stroke. Because the ovaries no longer produce estrogen, a progressive degenerative disease of the bone, osteoporosis, can set in. There are various ways to prevent bone loss, including good diet and exercise, and there are also treatments to reverse bone loss once it has started, usually some type of estrogen replacement. Hip fractures are a common result of osteoporosis in postmenopausal women, and this frequently leads to a cascade of events ending with death. Growing numbers of women in richer countries and the more affluent in the world's poorer countries are using hormone replacement therapy, hormonal medications to replace natural hormones lost due to menopause.

With the present low fertility rates around the world, women have the advantage of voluntarily reducing childbearing and the social benefits that this carries, but there are adverse biological consequences that science should be able to overcome. The modern woman has fewer children and lives longer. Consequently, she menstruates more often and spends many more years in the postmenopausal phase of life. These are biological differences that go along with a falling TFR. Unless we believe that women should return to the pattern of being constantly pregnant or lactating, we need to acknowledge that the present pattern of low fertility is here to stay and find acceptable means to counter the unwanted health risks and side effects associated with incessant ovarian cycles and menstruation. As it is now possible to counteract the debilitating effects of menopausal changes by the use of hormone replacement therapy, it will surely be possible to develop safe and acceptable methods to permit the woman of the twenty-first century to decide when she will have an ovarian cycle to establish a pregnancy and how to remain healthy and risk-free while benefiting from the health advantages of suppressing ovulation and menstruation for the remainder of her reproductive years.

It would be an ironic twist if the reduction of total fertility rates and the many social benefits this brings women and their families carries with it a new burden of illness for which modern science has no answers. Life-threatening afflictions such as childbed fever, once believed to be inevitable—"a woman's burden"—have been conquered by modern medicine. Science helped to bring about the revolution in fertility. Now science is called upon to reduce the legacy of risks to women's health and well-being that reproductive freedom carries.

4

The Pill and IUD Modernized Contraception

Human reproduction is regulated by a synchronized chain of events, each link dependent on the successful completion of the preceding one. We are constantly gaining a more detailed understanding of the process as scientists probe at more sophisticated levels of inquiry. A new generation of molecular biologists is unraveling the reproductive process, gene by gene, in order to improve diagnosis and treatment of reproductive disorders. Genes have been discovered that enable the egg to orchestrate the early events of sperm–egg interaction. Modern science has already improved the treatment of infertility, menopause-associated symptoms, and life-threatening diseases including breast cancer and osteoporosis. As we understand more about links in the reproductive chain of events, opportunities to advance contraceptive technology have also increased.

Whether you start with the Garden of Eden or elsewhere in humankind's time scale, it has usually been understood that sexual intercourse introduces the male factor responsible for fertilization. Noah's pairings for berths (and births) on his ark required a male and a female. Famous names in early science like Antonie van Leeuwenhoek, the seventeenth-century Dutch inventor of the microscope, believed that sperm contained preformed "little men." Much earlier, Galen, the court physician to the Roman Emperor Marcus Aurelius, thought the fallopian tube transported "female sperm" to the uterus from the ovary—should we say, "little women?"

Consequently, for centuries people attempted to prevent pregnancy by the simple and direct procedure of withdrawing the penis before ejaculation. This practice even gets a mention in the Old Testament. Linguistic scholars report that the practice of *coitus interruptus* has a slang name in virtually every tongue. In relatively recent times, mechanical barriers or chemicals introduced into the vagina in various formulations have been used. The sperm have been confronted with vulcanized roadblocks or plunged into creams, ointments, gels, foams, or effervescent fluids containing mercurial compounds, weak acids, soaps, or biological detergents. Strange concoctions used have ranged from crocodile dung in antiquity to Coca Cola in the twentieth century. Postcoital douching also became popular early in history. Australian aborigines include in the ceremony celebrating male puberty a ritualistic drilling of a hole in the base of the penis, using a sharpened twig to penetrate the urethra. The hole creates a fistula so the semen is diverted at the time of ejaculation. For urinating, the youth is taught to close the hole with a finger, in the manner of the flutist.

Contraceptive technology finally caught up with modernity when scientists turned their attention to the woman's ovulatory cycle and the hormonal control of reproduction in both sexes. The principle of periodic abstinence timed to avoid coitus near the day of ovulation was the first method of regulatory fertility that relied on evidence-based understanding of the reproductive process. That was in the 1920s when, independently, a Japanese scientist, Kyusaka Ogino and an Austrian, Herman Knaus, authored publications concluding that a woman should avoid sex around mid-cycle if she did not intend to become pregnant.

The Ogino-Knaus method was based on emerging understanding about the endocrinology of the ovarian cycle in women, establishing that ovulation occurs about 14 days before the first day of the next expected menstrual flow. Ogino and Knaus recognized that there is less variability in the last half of the cycle than in the first half, so that counting forward 14 days from the last expected period is an approximation of when to expect ovulation, but it could introduce predictive uncertainty. Ogino and Knaus understood when the egg is released, although they did not know how long it remained fertilizable and how long sperm survive in the fallopian tube. This knowledge came later when John Rock and Arthur Hertig made observations suggesting that the egg can be fertilized for about one day after it is released, and the sperm can wait around for roughly two days. Scientists have since upped the estimate for sperm so that now it is thought that the egg remains viable for one day and the sperm for six or seven days. The combination of unpredictability of the day of ovulation and the length of sperm survival causes uncertainty about the period of abstinence required. That the rhythm method did not prove to be as effective as other contraceptives does not detract from its historical importance as the first to be based on understanding the ovarian cycle.

It was several decades later before the necessary knowledge was marshaled to develop effective means to prevent ovulation medically, but when that moment came, the practice of contraception was revolutionized. The era of hormonal contraception was launched. The task was difficult. How could women maintain all the essential aspects of their reproductive endocrinology, except not release an egg, or by some other mechanism be protected from an unwanted pregnancy?

For a world that needs heroes who do not strum electric guitars or dunk basketballs, Dr. Gregory Pincus should have the recognition he deserves. In spite of many obstacles, he led the scientific effort that resulted in the first oral contraceptive, "the pill." If the Manhattan Project of the 1940s was the physicists' tour de force, the Worcester Project of the 1950s was one of the great achievements in reproductive biomedicine. Pincus was director of the Worcester Foundation for Experimental Biology in Massachusetts. His work may have been the single most important medical advance of the century for improving women's health.

Between 1960 and 2000, roughly 120 million women used the pill for a total of about 650 million years of woman-use. Assuming that without the pill, other methods of contraception would have been used, many with higher failure rates, countless unplanned and unwanted pregnancies would have occurred. Surveys show that about half would have ended in elective termination, many in countries where abortion was illegal and unsafe. This included most of the United States until 1973. The toll in terms of the death and injury to women would have been enormous. That's why I place the pill high on the list of titanic twentieth-century advances in women's health. The name Pincus should stand with Semmelweis in the history of medical progress for safe motherhood.

Pincus was a brilliant and imaginative scientist. When he told Margaret Sanger in 1951 that he believed that science was ready for developing an oral contraceptive, he had already broken new ground with his scientific work at Harvard. He had achieved in vitro fertilization of rabbit eggs, foreshadowing the later successes in assisted human reproduction, and he followed this with equally dramatic work on parthenogenesis. Screaming headlines about "test-tube babies" and "fatherless rabbits" elicited a storm of right-wing rage, laced with antiscience, antifeminism, and anti-Semitic attacks. That may have had something to do with Pincus's move to Clark University in Worcester, Massachusetts from sedate Harvard, where he failed to win tenure, in spite of his work being included in the university's list of greatest scientific achievements in its history, as part of its tercentenary celebration in 1936.

The twentieth century is sometimes called the American century. It was also the century of science. It brought an array of achievements that have changed our lives in ways that could not have been imagined. Think about the conversion from gaslight to electricity, from the horse and buggy to the modern automobile and air travel, the telephone, radio, and electronic communication, and the conquest of many diseases with drugs and vaccines. Consider also the exploration of space and the launching of satellites, the awesome power of nuclear fission, and of the minute silicon chip. Modern contraception stands with this list of scientific achievements that have guided the course of human history, particularly for its impact on the lives of women. Author Bernard Asbell was not mistaken when he entitled his 1995 book *The Pill: A Biography of the Drug That Changed the World.*

This does not mean that individual women gaining control over their own lives and fertility is simply a matter of the development of contraceptive methods. Technology is only part of the story along with social, cultural, and economic conditions and the motivation of individuals. Yet the development of new technology can contribute in a major way. It can provide methods that women and couples can voluntarily choose that are effective, safer, and more readily acceptable at any level of motivation. It's straightforward: good contraceptives are more likely to be used than bad contraceptives. That's true for any consumer product.

Before the pill and other modern methods, twentieth-century couples had a limited choice of contraceptive methods that were dismally ineffective for preventing conception. A 1935 survey revealed that contraceptive use in the United States was equally divided among the condom, douche, rhythm, and withdrawal. Failure rates must have been huge, forcing women to choose between high fertility or illegal and unsafe abortions in those pre-antibiotic years. The suffering this caused is what Margaret Sanger observed working as a nurse among poor immigrant women in lower Manhattan, inspiring her to start the birth control movement. She was convinced that more effective and more acceptable methods of contraception were urgently needed. This is what brought her to Worcester and to Gregory Pincus. Her friend and benefactor Katherine McCormick (heiress of the McCormick farm machine company) was also convinced that Pincus was the man who could deliver a perfect contraceptive that women could use safely, so she put up the money.

Pincus had attracted to the Worcester Foundation leaders in steroid biochemistry, reproductive biology, and related sciences. One crucial recruitment was Dr. M.C. Chang, a Cambridge University-trained physiologist known for his work on sperm physiology. At Worcester, Chang confirmed a previously neglected finding that injections of progesterone could suppress ovulation in laboratory animals. This was the observation that made it feasible to search for an oral contraceptive. Because progesterone was only weakly active when given orally, the problem became finding a related substance that could be taken by mouth and would act like progesterone.

Worcester was an exciting place in those years. Pincus's group always seemed to dominate our scientific meetings with startling new discoveries leading closer and closer to his goal. The Conference on Physiological Mechanisms Concerned with Conception was held at West Point, New York, in 1959. From around the world, scientists working on conception control assembled to present their work, but it was the Worcester studies on a possible oral contraceptive that everyone was eager to learn about.

Pincus had formed a liaison with the G.D. Searle Company of Illinois. The great strength of pharmaceutical companies that cannot be matched by academic institutions is large-scale chemical synthesis programs that can produce a stream of compounds which may have the potential for important biological activity. M.C Chang and his associate, Anne Merrill, devised imaginative animal tests to establish whether Searle's compounds possessed progesterone activity and found that some were super-progesterones. The active doses of these progestins were far lower than the dose of progesterone needed for similar activity. Furthermore, these compounds proved to be very potent when given orally to rabbits.

Next, it was necessary to test the best of the Searle compounds in women. Pincus collaborated with distinguished Harvard gynecologist Dr. John Rock, noted for his work in treating infertility. Rock had devised a treatment known as rebound therapy to treat women who had an infertility problem because they were only ovulating intermittently, if at all. They were given injections of high doses of progesterone to put the pituitary and ovaries at rest. After stopping treatment, the woman's natural hormone production would rebound to higher levels than before and stimulate ovulation. The treatment was modestly successful, but in those days there were no other choices. For Rock, access to orally active, super-progesterones was a promising way to improve treatment of his infertility patients. Rock and his young associates, Dr. Celso Ramon Garcia and Dr. Luigi Mastroianni, used the selected Searle drug, labeled SC4642, for advanced rebound therapy and were thrilled to find that they could confirm in women what Chang and Merrill had seen in laboratory animals. When word started to circulate among endocrinologists that women treated with SC4642 did not ovulate, the realization grew that an oral contraceptive was feasible. Would it be safe for women to use for years at a time? Would irregular menstrual-like bleeding be too difficult a side effect to overcome? Would the synthetic hormone cause masculinizing effects? Would a hormone used continuously by healthy women gain approval from the federal Food and Drug Administration? Questions like these dominated informal discussions and also came up at scientific meetings devoted to reproductive endocrinology.

The first trials of SC4642 to test the contraceptive effectiveness were started in April 1956, in Rio Piedras, Puerto Rico, under the supervision of Garcia and Dr. Edris Rice-Wray, medical director of Puerto Rico's Family Planning Association. Rice-Wray later told me that she had never heard of Pincus or Rock when the proposal was made to study the new oral contraceptive in Puerto Rico, but the demand for

effective birth control was so great among the women served by the
Family Planning Association that she didn't hesitate to agree. Garcia,
a devoted young doctor, was a rising star in obstetrics and gynecology.
At the time of the pioneering studies, he was an assistant professor at
the University of Puerto Rico. Naturally, his patients were Puerto Ri-
can, a fact overlooked by those who, through the years, have questioned why the early work was done on poor women in Puerto Rico.
Later in his career, long after the completion of the trials, Garcia was
a professor at the University of Pennsylvania. At his own expense, he
traveled down to Puerto Rico during his vacation time to provide annual physical exams and advice on any family medical problems to the
women who had been volunteers in those oral contraceptive studies
many years earlier. A second trial in Puerto Rico was begun in Hu-
macao, a year after the start of the Rio Piedras study. The confirmatory
trial was under the supervision of Adeline Pendleton (Penny) Satter-
thwaite, an obstetrician and gynecologist at a missionary hospital. Sat-
terthwaite was much loved by the women of the town, who referred
to her tenderly and affectionately simply as "la Doctora." The idea
that she would participate in the exploitation of the poor women of
Puerto Rico is laughable.

During early clinical trials, a product development issue arose that
proved to be critical. Before the world had heard of Enovid, the name
given to SC4642, Dr. I.C. Winter, medical director of the Searle Company, came to New York City with his company's scientific director,
Dr. Victor Drill, to consult with Dr. Warren Nelson, who was medical
director of the Population Council. I was Nelson's assistant, recently
recruited from Iowa to establish the council's laboratory at the Rockefeller Institute. (I was pleased to be included in the working lunch that
was arranged at Manhattan's fashionable East side restaurant, *Charles
à la Pomme Soufflé*. On my salary, that was not an everyday opportunity.) Winter and Drill wanted Nelson's advice on a matter that
had come up in manufacturing Enovid. During the synthesis of the
progesterone-like compound, norethynodrel, an estrogenic contami-
nant, 3-methyl-ethinyl estradiol, or mestranol, remained in each batch,
but the problem was that there was no consistency in the amount remaining from batch to batch. Therefore, Searle proposed to add an
amount of mestranol to each batch that would bring it up to a standard
quantity. So the original intent of Pincus and Rock to suppress ovulation with a synthetic progestin alone was to be changed, and Enovid

would become a combination of a progestin (norethynodrel) and an estrogen (mestranol). Pincus and Rock were part of the decision-making process and were in favor of the modification. They also believed, from the experience of the Boston gynecology group, that the combination would give better control of menstrual-like bleeding than a progestin alone. Winter was extremely impressed by this point and returned to it time and time again during the luncheon discussion. I wondered at the time if the Searle strategy was to emphasize the use of their product for "menstrual regulation" in case the idea of an oral contraceptive was greeted with a cold reception.

The question was posed to Nelson whether he thought the FDA would accept this modification of the study design, in midstream, so to speak? In the 1950s, the FDA did not have the rigorous requirements that it now has. Certainly, today you cannot even consider a change in dosage form, let alone add a new chemical component to an experimental medicine, unless you are willing to start all over again and study many issues, including possible results of drug interactions. But those were different times, and the FDA's procedures were less demanding. The agency did not, for example, have standing committees of experts for each subject in medicine as they do now. I've heard it said that if the pill were to be submitted for approval today, on the basis of the data then available, it probably would not be approved. I think that's true, not because the early work was sloppy or incomplete, but because FDA's requirements have grown more voluminous. It now takes a moving van to transport the documents needed to file a new drug application to the FDA headquarters in Rockville, Maryland.

I thought the *pommes soufflés* were overrated French fries; otherwise the meal was delicious and the conversation lofty and fascinating. It seemed to me to be a historical moment, discussing whether the first oral contraceptive the world would know would be a progestin only or a combination of progestin and estrogen. We were not aware at the time that nature had already made that decision, since (we now know) the woman's body naturally converts a small amount of norethynodrel back to its estrogenic precursor. In any event, Nelson concurred with the plan to add the mestranol, and Searle went ahead to create the world's first oral contraceptive as a combination pill (progestin plus estrogen) instead of a progestin alone, as originally envisioned by Pincus, Rock, and Sanger.

From the start, Searle was determined to market the product with an interrupted schedule of pill taking that would be 21 days on therapy and one week off therapy. The main purpose of this was the marketing decision that women would find it more acceptable to use a product that enabled them to be assured that they were not pregnant. If they were to take a pill continuously and have bleeding irregularities or not bleed at all (a certain percentage would be amenorrheic), they could have pregnancy anxiety. Drug-store pregnancy kits were still years away. Intermittent therapy would result in a menstrual-like bleeding after stopping the pill. It also seemed to the Searle executives to be more likely to win regulatory approval than a continuous-use product. Moreover, I think they did have in mind its use for menstrual regulation in case the oral contraceptive purpose faltered for medical, political, or religious reasons.

Searle was wise to seek Nelson's views at that point in their product development work. As president of the Endocrine Society, the country's most prestigious professional organization of endocrinologists, Nelson was likely to have a voice in the FDA's deliberations on a matter pertaining to hormonal contraception. At that time, the Parke-Davis Company of Detroit was also asking his advice in its efforts to develop another orally active progestin for use in gynecology, but not birth control. In a "Dear Doctor" letter sent to every U.S. physician, Parke-Davis had made it clear that the super-progesterone they had licensed from the Syntex Company of Mexico City and California, norethindrone, was not intended for birth control. We all knew by then that norethindrone, like norethynodrel, could suppress ovulation in women. Respected colleagues such as Roy Hertz at the National Institutes of Health in Bethesda, Maryland, and Edward Tyler, a fertility specialist in Westwood, California, had worked with the compound and had published scientific articles on its activity. Speculation at that time was that Parke-Davis, with a large hospital supplies division, was fearful of losing its large Catholic hospital business if they were identified with a birth control pill.

One stormy February day in 1956, Nelson had dispatched me to Detroit on his behalf for a meeting with Parke-Davis's endocrinologists, Dr. Dan McGinty and his colleagues, to review hormone assay results. Our laboratory had been studying the effects of norethindrone and other progestins on the testis as a possible approach to male contraception. What I most remember of that winter visit to the Midwest was that the returning flight, with its few foolhardy passengers on board, started in a hangar where the wings were deiced thoroughly before the pilot gunned the DC-6 out of the hangar for a dash to the runway, and off into the air before ice could build up again during the deluge of snow and sleet. The plane managed to fly; the use of progestins for male contraception never did.

Introduction of the pill launched the era of hormonal contraception, based on ovulation suppression using a combination of estrogen and progestin. It evolved to include the continuous use of a progestin alone, by oral administration, by injection, by a subdermal implant, a skin patch, and even by an intrauterine system.

More than 50 other products with different progestins, lower doses, and various schedules of administration have supplanted the original pill. Some products offer a change in the progestin dose over the month, attempting to mimic the hormonal levels of the ovarian cycle. The main change has been a significant decrease in the amounts of both hormones.

Margaret Sanger's dream became a reality, but the pill most women now use is vastly different from the original Pincus and Rock version that she and McCormick had the vision to sponsor, and the Syntex compound, eventually marketed as a contraceptive, initially by the Ortho division of the Johnson and Johnson Company and then, after a change of heart, by Parke-Davis and by Syntex itself. An October 20, 1998, a *New York Times* article about oral contraceptives on the fortieth anniversary of the pill reported. "This is not your mother's birth control pill." The article went on to say, "A major drop in the estrogen and progestin levels since the 1960's has made oral contraceptives safer and added several health benefits." The pill that most women use today is composed of different hormones. We are now into the third generation of progestins contained in the pill. It is a fraction—less than one-twentieth—of the original dose. Almost all of the prescriptions written today are for oral contraceptives containing much less estrogen than was present in the original formulations.

Our knowledge of the pill's biological effects is wide. The pill has been the subject of greater postmarketing surveillance for safety than any pharmaceutical product in history. A study published in 1999 in the *British Medical Journal* reported on 25 years of follow-up of more than 45,000 women who began their experience with the products using the original, high-dose oral contraceptives. Countless other studies have documented not only the safety but also the non-contraceptive health benefits of oral contraceptives: decreased risk of endometrial and ovarian cancer, decreased risk of colon cancer, decreased anemia, decreased dysmenorrhea, and maintenance of bone density. There is a reduction in the incidence of benign breast disease (cysts) with oral contraception use and no overall increased risk of breast cancer, but uncertainty remains regarding long-term use for those who start taking the pill when young. If there is an added risk, it appears to be small and may be offset by careful surveillance.

Although the constituents and dosage of the pill have changed, some features have stayed the same. These, too, are about to change. Since it was first introduced, the pill has been marketed as a three-week-on and one-week-off method. Consequently, during the off-week women usually have a false menstruation. This schedule was not a medical requirement, but a marketing decision based on the belief that women consider menstruation as natural, and would be reluctant to use a product that stopped their periods. It was also felt that gynecologists would be uneasy about losing vaginal bleeding as a diagnostic tool.

Over the years, some doctors have counseled women to take the pill continuously to avoid menstruation, both for convenience and for medical reasons. The first product designed for nonstop use of the pill (for three months at a time) has been given the green light by the FDA for final study and the company involved expects to place it (Seasonale) on the market by 2004. I believe that many nonstop pill products, for both contraception and menstruation control, will soon be available and widely used. Finally, women will be freed from the control of marketers who decided that women want to have a pseudo-menstruation every month. They'll be able to decide themselves.

Women will also have a wider choice of the hormones contained in oral contraceptive products. Currently, all brands use the original estrogens—ethinyl estradiol or its 3-methyl ether (mestranol). This is almost certain to change in coming years, with the development of so-called designer estrogens, compounds that give women specific benefits of estrogens without unwanted effects. This will increase confidence in the safety of oral contraceptives. And new products will provide additional non-contraceptive health benefits. We already have progestins that can help women improve their cholesterol profiles, and one that reduces water retention.

Dr. Carl Djerassi, a chemist involved in the synthesis of norethindrone, the pioneering Syntex compound, wrote 20 years before the end of the twentieth century that the birth control methods used in 2001 "will most likely be indistinguishable from those we have today." How to score his prediction's accuracy depends on definitions, but he was certainly right in foreseeing no major change in the mechanism of action on which contraceptive products for women are based. What Djerassi, or any of us for that matter, might not have predicted 20 years ago was that the most widely used reversible contraceptive by global count in 2001 would not be a pill, but the intrauterine device (IUD). American readers may find that surprising because the IUD has made little impact on contraceptive use in the United States, but the vast numbers who use it in China and its popularity in Europe and elsewhere are the reason it has moved to the top of the global list, with nearly 120 million users in the developing countries alone.

Modern IUD research began at about the same time that the final stages of research on oral contraceptives were in progress. To this day, we really can't say we understand why the presence of a foreign body in the uterus prevents pregnancy. We were particularly interested in learning whether it worked after fertilization, for we knew that would be important for some women to know. Using every test possible in modern science, we could not demonstrate the presence of fertilized eggs in IUD users, even when egg recovery studies were carried out. Mechanism of IUD action is a subject that was given high priority in my own laboratories both in New York and in New Delhi.

In the Indian studies with the large langur monkeys indigenous to north India, we found that the presence of an IUD reduced the number of sperm that reach the fallopian tubes where fertilization takes place. We confirmed this observation in our colony of rhesus monkeys in New York. One of the rhesus monkeys in these studies, a healthy and frisky female with a monkey-sized IUD in her uterus, escaped from her cage, near a window carelessly left open. We could not catch her easily because there was a new building going up on the Rockefeller University campus, and she had no trouble climbing the steel girders that were in place. Soon, she became very adept at snatching sandwiches from the construction crew's lunch boxes and running off with open cans of soda. The last monkey sighting on the Upper East Side of Manhattan led us to believe that she ended up as a pet for a dowager on Park Avenue.

The first modern IUD to undergo careful scientific scrutiny was designed by Dr. Jack Lippes, a Buffalo, New York, gynecologist. The

Lippes loop revived interest in a subject that had a politically tarnished past. When Austro-German medicine still enjoyed respect in the early 1930s, Dr. Ernst Graffenberg proposed to his gynecology colleagues in Leipzig that placing a small, flexible silver ring in the uterus could prevent pregnancy. Apparently hundreds of women had been using the Graffenberg ring by the time of his scientific report. Naziism was beginning to infest German professions, including medicine. According to Dr. Christopher Tietze, originally of Vienna, the fact that Graffenberg was a Jew influenced the scornful reception his report received. The overt criticism was that the ring would cause pelvic infection. Consequently, if it was mentioned in textbooks of gynecology up to the 1950s, it was only to condemn the Graffenberg ring as an instrument of potential harm. This was true even in the textbook edited by the noted Planned Parenthood advocate, Dr. Alan Guttmacher. When interest in IUDs first resurfaced in the 1960s, I searched the scientific literature and could not find a single report of even one case history of pelvic inflammatory disease associated with the use of the Graffenberg ring. It was clearly a case of guilt by misinformation.

Lippes' interest in the subject had been aroused by a scientific publication written by Dr. W. Oppenheimer, a physician who had worked with Graffenberg in Germany before surviving the Holocaust by immigrating to Palestine. Oppenheimer's publication had the wry title "The Lost Wedding Bands." It described his experience with patients in Israel who had fled Germany as young women and now, postmenopausal and living in Israel, had gynecological disorders requiring hysterectomy. In some surgically removed uteri, the pathologist unexpectedly found Graffenberg rings that had been so trouble-free through a lifetime of use that the women had totally forgotten that they had them. At about the same time, a Japanese doctor, Atsumi Ishihama, also reported no complications with long-term use of a similar IUD called the Ota ring.

In spite of the writings in his own textbook, Guttmacher advised the Population Council to look into intrauterine contraception in a serious, scientific manner. He had just returned from an around-the-world trip and was doubtful that a method that required taking a pill every day would have much impact in the world's poorest and underprivileged countries. He thought the need for a long-acting method was greater.

As I read tables on contraceptive use around the world in the year

2000, I realize how prescient Guttmacher's advice was 40 years ago. He urged us to sponsor a meeting so that current information could be reviewed. The meeting was held in New York. Oppenheimer, Ishihama, Tietze, and Guttmacher attended. We learned that Lippes was not the only gynecologist inspired to design a linear plastic IUD that could easily be inserted without dilating the cervix. The outcome of the meeting was that the Population Council set up a comparative study of several IUDs, organized and supervised by Tietze, with an advisory committee that included Guttmacher and several other professors of gynecology.

For at least 15 years, from 1962 to 1977, the Population Council provided substantial grant funds to investigators in many countries to study the effectiveness, safety, and mechanism of action of IUDs. The choice of an acronym for intrauterine device was not a routine decision. Tietze did not like the term "IUD" because in obstetrics, the initials were already used to indicate "intrauterine death." In our advisory committee, we agreed on "IUCD", referring to "intrauterine contraceptive device," but we quickly learned that space-stingy medical journals usually edited it down to the shorter version. So, despite our best efforts, "IUD" became general usage, at least in the United States.

By the time the Lippes loop entered the market in 1965, it was by far the most extensively and carefully tested contraceptive product in history. More than 10,000 women had participated in trials in 10 countries. The Indian experience was particularly eventful. Colonel Raina, India's Director of Family Planning, had sent a file to the Health Minister, Dr. Sushila Nayar. Nayar was the famous Indian physician who had accompanied Mahatma Gandhi as his personal doctor on his march to the sea protesting the salt tax imposed by India's British rulers. There had been no response from the Minister, and, until her permission was granted, Raina was reluctant to authorize the first IUD trials in India.

As the colonel's advisor, I was aware of this while eagerly awaiting the go-ahead to begin the study at two hospitals in New Delhi and elsewhere in India. Learning that Nayar, a graduate of the Johns Hopkins School of Public Health in Baltimore, Maryland, would have a stopover in Los Angeles on a trip to a women's conference in Mexico City, I cabled (in those pre–e-mail, pre-telefax days) Guttmacher suggesting that he, a revered Baltimorean, meet her in Los Angeles and explain the extensive testing that had already taken place around the world. When Nayar returned to India she forwarded the approved file with a hand-written note saying that the illustrious Dr. Alan Guttmacher had flown all the way from New York to the West Coast to tell her about IUDs. That was good enough for her. Raina and I were elated.

The timing was perfect because my colleague, Dr. Anna Southam, was returning to India from a short visit to New York, and she could carry the IUDs for the study with her luggage. I met her plane at Delhi's Palam airport and was dismayed that the carton carrying IUDs did not appear at the baggage claim. Pan Am Flight 1 was being readied for the next leg of its around-the-world flight. With the cooperation of the airport public health officer, who recognized me from his studies at the All India Medical Institute, we were able to commandeer a vehicle and dash out to the plane before the cargo doors were closed. We persuaded a baggage handler to go back into the compartment and search for an overlooked box destined for Delhi. To happy grins all around, he reappeared at the hatch opening, holding the small carton that almost had continued an around-the world flight, hidden behind other cargo. By this time our antics had attracted the attention of the customs officials who wanted to know what was in the box. "Family Planning!" I declared, and we passed without further question.

The initial international trials with the Lippes loop had been carried out in Taiwan and South Korea, so by that the time Indian studies began, it was the major contraceptive technology used in the family planning programs of those countries. As scientific credibility grew, thanks to Tietze's well-documented study, more and more countries around the globe adopted the method.

I was sorry to see that its popularity aroused competitive anxieties in commercial companies that pioneered the marketing of oral contraceptives and were eager to expand the use of their products in the family planning programs of developing countries. In Mexico, a Syntex consultant attempted to stigmatize IUDs by labeling them "abortos plasticos" (plastic abortions), though fully aware that they do not work by causing abortions. One egregious case was a sudden spate of press reports that IUD insertions had been responsible for an epidemic of hepatitis in South Korea. This came as a shock to us in New York because we had a Population Council office in Seoul and I was constantly in touch with the president of the Korean Planned Parenthood Association, Dr. Jae Moo Yung, and not a single case of hepatitis had ever been reported. The same was true in Taiwan where monitoring untoward events was my laboratory's responsibility. The reports eventually fizzled because the hepatitis cases proved to be nonexistent.

Years later, a friend sent me a memorandum given to him inadvertently from the files of the G.D. Searle Company. It was from one of their foreign sales representatives who was organizing a Bombay meeting on contraception at about the time of the hepatitis hoax. It read, "I think I've got the issue that can kill the IUD. At tomorrow's meeting, a Korean doctor will claim that the inserter spreads hepatitis." My friend, General Bill Draper, a strong supporter of family planning, found the memo accidentally included in a stack of clippings and other papers given to him by Searle's president to support his complaint that the Population Council was opposing the introduction of oral contraceptives in family planning programs. I believe this misconception was prompted by a speech I had given in Los Angeles in which I calculated that if India had to pay the bill itself, the cost of the pill for the likely number of users in the country at that time would have absorbed India's entire foreign exchange budget for the import of all medical and hospital supplies. That was fact, not just spin.

In addition to Pincus, I have another candidate for unsung hero of women's health—Christopher Tietze. His meticulous work, together with his wife Sarah Lewit, in organizing and managing the initial comprehensive IUD studies, had many important outcomes. In all countries, it strengthened the will of health officials to initiate family planning efforts because they felt there was a technology available that they could afford and that they could believe in. His work proved that IUDs are effective and safe. It prompted research to find even better IUDs.

Tietze was also a women's health hero in another battle. His epidemiological studies on abortion proved critical when the Supreme Court ruled on *Roe vs. Wade* in 1973. In Justice Blackmun's majority opinion, he cites Tietze's work in analyzing the health risks and benefits of termination at different stages of pregnancy.

The Lippes loop and other plastic IUDs of the 1960s were extremely effective compared to other contraceptive methods, but the real breakthrough on effectiveness occurred when copper-releasing IUDs were developed. This started as a small laboratory research project with rabbits, by Dr. Jaime Zipper in Santiago, Chile, funded by the Population Council. As with IUDs more generally, we don't understand why the release of copper in the uterus is so effective in preventing pregnancy.

There is evidence from animal studies that the copper ions released from the copper wire attached to the plastic IUD act to stop most sperm before they reach the fallopian tube, but there are probably other mechanisms of action, as well, to account for the high level of effectiveness in preventing pregnancy.

In spite of the fact that the miniscule amount of copper released each day is about equivalent to the copper content of a portion of cooked spinach, we undertook extensive studies to establish the safety, first in animals and then in women, of copper release within the uterus. We sought the advice of a leading expert on Wilson's disease, a rare condition caused by the deposition of copper in the joints, and his reassurance later proved important when the FDA decided to treat the copper-releasing IUD not as a device but as a drug, requiring the same safety and effectiveness studies demanded of a new pharmaceutical product in order to be given approval.

Intrauterine contraception suffered a severe setback in the United States when the Dalkon Shield was put on the market by the A.H. Robins Company. By the time it was withdrawn, several deaths had been ascribed to the Dalkon Shield, an IUD that never should have been marketed in the first place. Personally, I sided with the plaintiffs in the litigation against the Dalkon Shield. Our IUD advisory committee had declined to accept for inclusion in our multiple device comparative study the earlier version of the Dalkon Shield on the grounds of its potential health hazards to users. The Robins Company was aware of our decision before they acquired rights to the device from gynecologist Hugh Davis and proceeded with the development and marketing of the Dalkon Shield. Unfortunately, this tragic episode had a negative impact on all IUDs in the U.S. market.

The copper T-380A is the most effective of copper-bearing IUDs; it is about equal in effectiveness to surgical sterilization. The copper T-380A was developed through research sponsored by the Population Council. It was initially marketed by the G.D. Searle, along with a variation of the original design, known as the Copper 7.

Within months after the giant chemical corporation, Monsanto, acquired Searle in 1985, both IUD products were pulled from the market. My friend Dr. Howard Schneiderman was vice president for research at Monsanto at that time, and his wife was active in the local Planned Parenthood affiliate in California where they lived. Schneiderman, a talented endocrinologist who had made major discoveries in the field of insect hormones, had been professor of biology at the University of California at Irvine before joining Monsanto. On his invitation, I had been a visiting professor at Irvine and gave a series of lectures, including a description of our IUD research. He was, therefore, aware of our involvement in the development of copper-releasing IUDs.

After the product withdrawal, he called me to explain that the reason for this decision was the mounting cost of defending lawsuits against all IUDs stemming from the litigation against the Dalkon Shield. There was an army of litigating lawyers out there, experienced in winning Dalkon Shield cases, eager to identify new targets. Monsanto was unwilling to expose the entire assets of the corporation for the sake of products which, though medically safe, were vulnerable to litigation while adding little to total corporate revenues.

Ortho Pharmaceuticals (now Ortho-MacNeil) of New Jersey, which also distributed a copper T-IUD, followed Monsanto out of the U.S. market. Consequently, IUDs virtually disappeared from the United States for several years, until a small company was formed to market the copper T-380A. With such limited distribution and marketing, relatively few American women use IUDs. Now that the product has been reacquired by Ortho-MacNeil, a company with excellent experience in the marketing of contraceptives, this is beginning to change.

Intrauterine contraception, using the same products that were withdrawn from women in the United States, is the method of choice in many other countries, representing a range of different cultures. Intrauterine devices are used by 30% of contracepting women in Sweden and Norway and by more than half of all couples using reversible contraception in China, Cuba, Turkey, and Vietnam. Its appeal is based on simplicity of use, ease of reversibility, absence of medical side effects, low cost, and remarkable effectiveness. In a seven-year study, the World Health Organization found that the contraceptive effectiveness of the Copper T-380A is equal to that of surgical sterilization. The device maintains its effectiveness for 10–12 years. It can be realistically described as reversible sterilization.

A Copper T-380A IUD can be manufactured and sold profitably for about $1. It's hard to imagine improving on this cost for the amount of effective contraception provided. Yet, the biting irony is that many insurance company prescription drug plans do not include contraceptives in their coverage—but they will reimburse for Viagra. I have a slide that I show in lectures that says: "Insurance Company Logic: $10 for 1 erection—we'll pay; $1 for 10 years of contraception—we won't pay." There is a message in there about attitudes toward women's health.

Another intrauterine contraceptive system popular in European countries for several years has been introduced in the United States. This is the levonorgestrel-releasing intrauterine system. It is as effective as the Copper T-380A and women have fewer days of vaginal bleeding than can be expected when using a copper IUD. The Copper T-380A has at least a 10-year life span; the levonorgestrel-releasing intrauterine system, marketed under the trade name Mirena, lasts for five years.

The pill and the IUD were the giant steps in contraceptive technology that began in the 1950s. By the century's end it was clear that they filled different niches in the world's contraceptive portfolio. The pill had become a $2.5 billion industry, primarily in richer countries and among the growing middle class of developing countries. The IUD rose to the top of the list of reversible contraceptives in use, primarily because it was brought into the national family planning programs of several governments, including China. Many countries became familiar with the method through the participation of their doctors in the large international studies sponsored by the Population Council.

As for China's priority on IUD use, I can only speculate. Surely the People's Republic of China was monitoring events in Taiwan, which had excellent experience with the original Lippes loop and subsequent generations of IUDs. The American writer, Edgar Snow, came to see me in 1964, during the years of the tightly closed bamboo curtain. He told me that he was going to visit China and Vice Premier Chou En Lai had asked him to bring news about modern contraception in the West. This was not surprising, since China watchers at that time knew there was a struggle going on about population policy, with military leaders opposed to government sponsored birth control and Chou En Lai quietly supporting it. As Snow and I conversed, I rummaged through an untidy desk drawer, came up with a sealed plastic bag of newly manufactured copper T IUDs, and gave them to him. In return, he gave me an autographed copy of his book, *The Other Side of the River*, which I still cherish. Some months later, I had a letter from Switzerland. "Dear Sheldon," it read, "The IUDs you fished out of your desk are now in a drawer in the desk of Comrade Chou!" Perhaps they stayed in that secure storage place during the dark days of the Cultural Revolution, waiting until the proper moment to move ahead with a plan to implement government support for family planning. When I was taken to see health clinics in China in 1977, after the Cultural Revolution, a highlight of each visit was showing me the copper T IUDs manufactured in China, complete with a Mandarin language translation of the package insert of the devices carried to China by Edgar Snow.

5

Beyond the Pill and the IUD

After the pill and the IUD, it would be 30 years before a totally new method of contraception gained approval by the FDA. This was the subdermal implant system, Norplant. Like the pill, its primary action is based on the inhibition of ovulation; like the IUD, it is long-acting, reversible, and has an effectiveness in the range of surgical sterilization. Because it lasts for 5 years, one visit to a clinic can replace 1800 days of pill-taking. Because it does not require a gynecological procedure, it offers a new choice for long-term contraception.

Implant contraception began in my New York laboratory, but was possible only because others had made important discoveries. We were attempting to develop a removable plug for reversible closure of the vas deferens in men. The rabbit was our animal model, and the material we were using was Silastic, a Dow-Corning medical-grade plastic. The actual chemical name is polydimethyl siloxane. It is the polymerized form of a silicone-based compound. The idea was to take advantage of its biocompatibility: It could be used in the human body without causing a reaction or allergic response. When we started this work, Silastic had already been in medical use for over 15 years. One major application was slender tubing used to drain fluid accumulating around the brain into the abdominal cavity for children born with hydrocephalus. This same tubing would ultimately be used for manufacturing Norplant. We had done extensive literature reviews to assure that Silastic was safe.

Occasionally, a Dow-Corning representative, Silas Braley, would stop by to see how our research was coming along. He would usually meet with Dr. Ken Laurence, who was in charge of the reversible vasectomy project. On one such occasion, Ken was out of town so I met with Braley. He mentioned that he had just visited a pediatric surgeon who used silastic in experimental surgery, Dr. Judah Folkman at Children's Hospital in Boston, who later became even better known for his work with angiogenesis inhibitors for cancer treatment. Folkman and his colleague, Dr. David Long, Braley told me, discovered that oil-soluble dyes slowly diffuse out of Silastic. I immediately thought, if oil-soluble dyes, why not oil-soluble hormones? Putting this together with biocompatibility, I could envisage a system placed subdermally, like the hydrocephalus shunts, that would slowly release a steroid hormone and serve as a long-acting contraceptive: An "under-the-skin-pill," as one of my young daughters would describe it at some future date when her teacher asked the pupils to tell what their fathers did.

That same afternoon I started preliminary experiments in white laboratory rats and in a matter of days realized that this could work. I chose to test the idea using an estrogen because it was easy to measure its effects in female rats. This could hardly be considered useful as a contraceptive. When I tried progesterone, which might have been a candidate, it leached out from the Silastic so quickly that the effect was over in just a few days. None of this could not happen today because animal experiments, like studies involving people, have to be written up carefully, justifying why and how many animals have to be used, and submitted to an institutional review board for approval. It can take months.

There was much to do ahead. The compound used would have to be potent enough so that a tiny amount released each day would be enough to act as a contraceptive. The form of the implant would have to be suitable for human use. The amount stored would have to last long enough to make the implant practical.

Meanwhile, Dr. Jorge Martinez-Manatou of Mexico City published a paper in a medical journal showing that a progestin-only pill taken every day can be an effective contraceptive. The pill he studied was a low dose of the Syntex super-progesterone, norethindrone. The method quickly was dubbed "the mini-pill." This was an encouraging development, for we realized that if we could identify the right super-progesterone, our subdermal implant would also work. In fact, we theorized, it might be more effective because we could achieve a more constant blood level than the ups and downs of daily pill-taking. Martinez-Manatou was the Syntex consultant mentioned in chapter 4 who labeled IUDs "abortos plasticos" in an attempt to discredit them in Catholic Mexico. Nevertheless, we formed a close friendship that endures to this day. Incidentally, Martinez-Manatou later became the effective and successful head of Mexico's Women's Health and Family Planning program.

At some point, I invited one of the postgraduate fellows in the laboratory to join the project. This was an important decision because Dr. Horacio Croxatto of Santiago, Chile, became a vital addition to the project. He played an active role in the New York experiments and ultimately presented a report of our work at an annual meeting of the American Fertility Society before he returned to Chile, where he continued to work on the idea. Others in the lab lent their expertise for needed skills such as radioactive steroid determinations, hormone assays, implant design, and animal studies. As in all scientific developments, years of effort by many people followed that initial meeting with Silas Braley.

The development of subdermal implants also took the cooperation of some key individuals in other organizations. One was Folkman, whose patent on the principle of steroid diffusion through Silastic had been assigned to the Dow-Corning Company of Midland, Michigan. He willingly agreed to waive royalty rights for any product that might come out of the Population Council's work. At one point his lawyer thought that the council should pay for this right, but Folkman quickly vetoed that suggestion because of his respect for our work around the world. At Dow-Corning, Ira Hutchinson, a high-level executive, needed to approve of the waiving of rights. He knew nothing about the Population Council and our humanitarian mission, so it took a few visits to New York before he understood that we were not intending to use their patent for commercial purposes. On one of the visits, Hutchison's wife, Eunice, who was active in Midland's pro-life community, accompanied him, and she left New York after dining with my wife and me realizing that our devotion to the well-being of children matched her own. Hutchison had forewarned me that her reaction would be a bell-wether to the reaction of many others at Dow-Corning and in Midland.

Ultimately, we received the waivers needed to justify the major investment that would be required, knowing that we would have access to the appropriate intellectual property rights on Silastic to carry an implant method to completion and marketing for public sector use. We would have to worry about the same issue when the appropriate progestin was selected, since all the candidate compounds we were testing were the property of one company or another.

It soon became evident that the task of finding the optimal contraceptive compound and the ideal form of the method would be lengthy and complicated. Instead of hiring a large clinical research group, as was customary for product development efforts in pharmaceutical companies, I decided to form a team of talented people who would stay in their home academic positions and work with us on contraceptive development projects. This needed major financial support, so I presented the idea at a Bellagio Conference on Population at the Rockefeller Foundation's Conference and Study Center in Bellagio, Italy. This was one of a series of high-level conferences that influenced the agenda for population-funding policy within foundations and international assistance agencies. It was at these conferences, for example, that the United Nations Development Program was advised to initiate the U.N. Fund for Population Activities (UNFPA); the World Bank was encouraged to add a program on population and health to its portfolio of activities; and the World Health Organization received the recommendation to start a program on human reproduction research. Bellagio conferences were also instrumental in major events in other aspects of international development. It was in the same meeting room some years earlier that the plans were laid and funding pledged for the network of international agricultural research centers that gave birth to the "Green Revolution."

When my turn came, the conferees included the director general of the World Health Organization, president of the World Bank, directors of the United Nations special programs UNICEF, UNFPA, and UNDP (United Nations Development Programme), and senior officers of the major U.S. foundations. I made my presentation on a day when I was suffering from jet lag and was a bit under the weather, but it won their support—thanks in large measure to my Ford Foundation supporters, Oscar "Bud" Harkavy and David Bell. Bell had joined the foundation with McGeorge Bundy after both had served in the Kennedy and Johnson administrations. Harkavy had launched and directed the Ford Foundation's important program in population. He appreciated the importance of both basic and applied research to bring about technological advances. We used to say admiringly that Harkavy knew more reproductive biology than any other economist. Another important supporter on that exciting day was Robert S. McNamara, president of the World Bank.

With the financial support assured, I traveled around the world to describe the idea to doctors I thought we should include. Some were friends who had worked in my laboratory at some time, others were names I knew from the scientific literature whose work seemed to me to be appropriate for what we wanted to accomplish. This group became the International Committee for Contraception Research (ICCR) which, over the years, became a major success story in the field of contraceptive and reproductive health product development and continues to do outstanding work. John Ross, at The Future's Group, calculated that in the year 2000, products developed by the Population Council's ICCR since its inception in 1971 accounted for 50.9% of reversible methods used in the developing countries. More than 120 million women in the developing world were using its products.

The initial members included physician/scientists from Austria (Julian Frick), Brazil (Elsimar Coutinho), Chile (Anibal Faundes), Finland (Tapani Luukkainen), Sweden (Elof Johansson), and the United States (Daniel Mishell, Jr.). Each was either an obstetrician/gynecologist or urologist and each had, in addition, a specialized nonclinical talent such as epidemiology, reproductive biology, or hormone biochemistry. At the first meeting, I presented the early information we had gathered, and the ICCR agreed to include implant contraception on the list of feasible leads to pursue. One of the group's first undertakings was an extensive search for the optimal contraceptive hormone to serve as the active ingredient of an implant. At first, we decided on a progestin called megestrol acetate, which was licensed to us by the British Drug House (BDH) of the United Kingdom. After we had made considerable progress with this product as the basis for a contraceptive implant, it was suddenly withdrawn by BDH because of adverse findings when tested in beagle dogs. It was a discouraging setback, but we continued the project. Next, we tested all progestins being used for oral contraceptives or for other gynecological purposes. A major advance in the chemistry of super-progesterones provided us with a vital assist. Until the early 1970s all progesterone-like hormones used for contraception were synthesized from natural precursor materials of either animal or plant origin. Then a British chemist announced a process of total synthesis to create a progestin named norgestrel, and this began the second generation of orally active progestins used in contraceptives.

For our implant project, the exciting feature of norgestrel was its high potency per unit weight compared to other progestins. The same capsule volume could hold more hormone potency than possible with other compounds. And it was a stroke of luck when we discovered in the laboratory that the compound's diffusion characteristics from Silastic were the best for our purposes of the many compounds we tested. This meant both a reduction in the number of capsules required to achieve a steady-state blood level that would stay above the threshold needed for contraceptive action and a prolongation of the time that capsules could remain effective as a contraceptive.

Ultimately our choice came down to two compounds, norgestrel, then licensed to the Wyeth Corporation of Radnor, Pennsylvania, and another super-progesterone we had received from the Roussell-UCLAF Company of Paris, France. Its code name was R2010 (no relation to RU486, about which you will read more later). This company had an excellent steroid synthesis program headed by Dr. Edouard Sakiz, a friend whom I knew from the time he was in the laboratory of Professor Robert Courrier, a pioneer in progesterone research.

The final selection of norgestrel came after a comparative study undertaken in Brazil, Chile, Denmark, Finland, the Dominican Republic, and Jamaica. Implants with the Wyeth compound produced a higher level of contraceptive effectiveness; the Rousell compound excelled in limiting the amount of vaginal bleeding. I wanted to continue developing both products so that women could have the option of choosing the quality they preferred, but budgetary constraints forced us to make a choice. Sakiz was disappointed (and miffed) when we decided that effectiveness was the more important consideration. He is an imaginative and entrepreneurial executive who relished the idea of scooping the major pharmaceutical companies with the first implant contraceptive. We overcame that disagreement and continue our friendship, I'm glad to say.

Selection of norgestrel meant that we needed to negotiate an agreement with Wyeth for a supply of the compound and for the right to use their patented compound for our novel purpose. Ordinarily, companies are reluctant to release compounds that are used in their successful commercial products for other uses. An unexpected finding could be extremely damaging. By this time, Wyeth's line of oral contraceptives was the high-riding leader of the pack in the United States, so there was a lot at stake. Once again, the credit belongs to an in-house executive who believed in the importance of the Population Council's work. At Wyeth, it was Dr. Richard Bogash, a chemist with a worldly view, who had risen to become a vice president of the company. He persuaded his company to enter into an "agreement to agree" with the Population Council so that we could proceed with our implant studies with assurance that, if successful, a product would be made available to women around the world.

It sounds so straightforward in retrospect, but we hit brick walls along the way. On at least two occasions I can recall, we came close to dropping the whole idea. We had already abandoned the goal of developing an implant for men. Early findings convinced us that the obstacles were too great to overcome. Primarily, this was because there was no androgenic hormone available having the high potency characteristic that would make it suitable for use as a subdermal implant. Years later the ICCR located such a compound and picked up the male implant idea once again.

Before the good fortune of norgestrel, we were studying progestins of weaker potency, and the number of implants women would require to obtain adequate blood levels for ovulation suppression was becoming more and more impractical with each trial. The brunt of this problem was being borne by Coutinho in Brazil. Initially, he was the ICCR coordinator of the clinical implant studies and became the target of attack from politically motivated groups who criticized him for accepting financial support from the United States. Fortunately, the dean of his medical school backed him in what was becoming a nasty situation in his hometown of Salvador, Bahia.

Within the ICCR, opinions differed about the potential and merits of the leads we were pursuing. When we were meeting in Austria, in the picturesque Alpine town of Igls, overlooking Innsbruck, I had a bad respiratory infection and stayed in bed while the ICCR meeting proceeded without me. In my absence, Elsimar had to stage a filibuster to keep the group from voting on discontinuing the implant project. It was a question of priority in the allocation of scarce funds, not disagreement on effectiveness or safety. It would have been a close vote. We persevered.

Over the course of our work, more than 50,000 women in 44 countries took part in various investigations. Some 400 articles were published in peer-reviewed scientific journals. We tried to get an answer to any question that came up or any safety issue that someone could hypothesize. We looked for and found no clinically significant changes in liver, kidney, pancreas, adrenal, or thyroid function. No change in bone density could be measured. There was no rise in total cholesterol or shift in ratio of good and bad cholesterol. Many studies around the world found that Norplant doesn't cause an elevation in blood pressure.

Despite the fact that users can experience extra days of menstrual-like bleeding and spotting, blood iron and hemoglobin levels are not decreased. In fact, among women who have low hemoglobin levels to begin with, after a year of Norplant use, iron levels increase because overall blood loss is less than that of normal menstruation. This is one of the non-contraceptive health benefits that our research disclosed. Women who had previously suffered from severe menstrual cramps or excessive bleeding, dysmenorrhea, or menorrhagia found relief while using Norplant. When questioned about their complaints or satisfaction with the method at the time of renewal of implants for a second five-year period of use, these benefits often came up along with satisfaction about the security of the method's contraceptive effectiveness.

The World Health Organization has completed a postmarketing surveillance of Norplant under normal conditions of everyday use in eight countries. This massive and expensive effort followed roughly 8000 Norplant users for 5 years and compared their health records to 8000 women who used either IUDs or sterilization. This unprecedented study of the safety of a contraceptive method gave Norplant a sweeping bill of health with respect to major diseases. No significant excess of cancer or cardiovascular events, such as stroke, heart attack, or blood clots was observed in women using Norplant compared to the others. In two of the eight countries involved in the study (China and Chile), there was an increase in the incidence of transient gall bladder disease. This did not appear in the other six countries. Contrary to earlier studies, there was an apparent tendency toward blood pressure increase in some centers. The study design may have been responsible because the measurements were taken as the women were waiting to have their implants removed.

In addition to the World Health Organization, many American and international professional organizations have undertaken detailed reviews of the efficacy and safety of Norplant and have endorsed its use. This list includes the American College of Obstetricians and Gynecologists and the American Society for Reproductive Medicine.

Norplant was introduced in the United States in 1991. It consists of 6 flexible, silicone-based capsules, each containing 36 milligrams of levonorgestrel (a more potent version of the original norgestrel). The material used for the tubing was identical to that sold by Dow-Corning for earlier medical devices. The tubing-wall thickness, which controls the rate of diffusion, was specified on the basis or our research and custom manufactured for Norplant. The implants release the drug into the circulation at a relatively constant rate over five years. Marketing began much earlier in Europe. Finland was the first country to give approval in 1984. Sweden approved Norplant in 1985, the same year that International Planned Parenthood Federation of London included Norplant on the list of contraceptive commodities made available to its affiliates throughout the world. By the time of FDA approval, nearly 5 million women around the world had used Norplant.

When the United States joined in, Norplant became essentially a globally available method. There were exceptions and, unfortunately, Brazil was one. The reason has nothing to do with uncertainty about safety or effectiveness of the method. Ironically this turned not on the earlier, politically motivated Salvador criticisms but another political skirmish when a new administration's Health Ministry officials sought to criticize and undo the actions taken by a previous administration.

The details illustrate how a scientific undertaking can become entangled in political infighting. It happens all too frequently in the field of contraception and fertility regulation. Dr. Anibal Faundes, a professor at the University of Campinas, Brazil, and an original ICCR member, designed a field trial of Norplant in Brazil. The protocol was crystal clear with respect to the ethics of studies involving human subjects. It specified the number of cases, the features of the study that protected the rights of participants, informed consent, peer review—all of the features one would expect of Faundes, a person with high ethical standards.

During the ICCR deliberations, it was usually Faundes who raised the ethical considerations for every step we took. In Brazil, after Health Ministry clearance and once the study got underway, additional Brazilian hospitals wanted to participate, so Faundes requested approval of an amendment, increasing the number of cases, a step that many clinical investigators would not even bother to take. He waited and waited for a reply and finally wrote to the ministry saying that, unless he heard otherwise, he would assume there was no objection and the new cases would be included. The continuing silence from officialdom became tacit approval, so he added the new cases under the same tight controls of the original protocol. This is what the new administration officials attacked. They closed the entire study on the grounds that it was going on without proper authorization. The losers were the women of Brazil where, in Salvador, much of the pioneering work on implant contraception had been done.

Everyone was impressed with the effectiveness of the method. Our Norplant development studies revealed pregnancy rates during the first five years averaging 0.2 per hundred woman-years of use. This exceeds by far the levels of protection against pregnancy achieved with other reversible methods. One way to think about it is that if 500 women use it for one year, there will be 1 unplanned pregnancy. For pill users the total number would be 10 times higher. Users of diaphragm, withdrawal, or rhythm would have method failures of roughly 20 per 100 per year. Couples using no contraception could expect to have pregnancies at the rate of about 85 per 100 per year.

Continuation-of-use rate is another measure of the success of a method of contraception. This is determined by answering the question, if 100 women start to use the method at the beginning of a year, how many are continuing to use it at the end of the year? Continuation rates are high for Norplant compared, for example, to the pill. Some subgroups of pill users can reach the 50% discontinuation point within the first year of use. On the other hand, two-thirds of Norplant users continued to use the method after 5 years in our own long-term studies. Over 90% completed five years of use in the World Health Organization study. In part, the successful continuation rate is a function of the method's clinic dependency. While an oral contraceptive user will discontinue because she runs out of her supply of pills or simply decides to stop, a Norplant user who wants to discontinue must take the positive step of going to a clinic to have the implant removed. This feature places an ethical responsibility on providers to assure that women always have access to facilities where trained personnel are available and are prepared to offer removals on demand.

Two independent studies done in Philadelphia and Baltimore illustrate this point. They were carried out by university-affiliated hospitals with teen pregnancy programs. The United States has the highest teen pregnancy rate of any industrialized country. It is twice as high as in Sweden and four times as high as the rate in the Netherlands. For an American teenager, it is the second baby that brings most disruption to her life, frequently compelling her to drop out of school and become welfare dependent. Among young teenagers, one out of three is likely to have a second baby within two years after the first child. In the studies I mentioned, the young mothers who had just given birth to their first child were given, in addition to abstinence counseling, a choice of Norplant, the pill, or condom use. Nearly two years later, 19 out of a 100 of the pill users had an unwanted second pregnancy, even more unwanted pregnancies occurred in the condom group, and in the Norplant group there was just 1 pregnancy. The pregnancy involved a young woman who asked to have the implants removed and, although given counseling on other methods, failed to start another method and became pregnant.

As the data were pouring in from studies around the world, the method was being called reversible sterilization, and that was a good characterization. This is significant in cultures where surgical or permanent methods of sterilization are forbidden but reversible methods are not. When a country study was planned for Egypt, my friend Dr. Fouad Hefnawi, who had been in our laboratory when the Silastic diffusion work started, asked me to join him to visit the grand imam of Al Azhar Mosque in Cairo, seat of the oldest and most authoritative Muslim university in the world. His approval was essential. As we entered his suite of offices, I was overwhelmed by the magnificent furnishings and rugs, but uncertain if I would have answers to his questions. The imam listened intently as I explained Norplant. He asked me only one question. "Is it reversible?" I assured him that it was. Permission was granted.

Approval followed in other Muslim countries including Indonesia, where implant contraception quickly became popular. I have never understood this fully and have always been skeptical of the explanation given by anthropologist friends that under-skin adornments are a part of Indonesian culture so that this approach to contraception seemed perfectly understandable in that country. I thought it probably had to do with the emphasis placed on the method in the Health Ministry's program. In fact, it worried me that they were placing too much emphasis on Norplant before clinic personnel were adequately trained for the insertion and removal procedures.

On a trip to Bali when the Indonesian Norplant program was well underway, I was invited to meet the local health officials. I expected questions about Norplant removal techniques and thought that this would be the main subject of discussion. It was, until the Indonesian doctors and nurses realized that one of my accompanying colleagues was Elsimar Coutinho whose research had launched the first 3-month injectable contraceptive, DepoProvera. They had been using it for years and were thrilled to meet its inventor.

An original member of the ICCR, Coutinho was also a founding member of another reproductive health product-development program, called South-to-South Cooperation in Reproductive Health. All its members were from developing countries, a concept that was based on the belief that these colleagues had mutual problems and experience so that they could constructively learn from each other. The initial executive director was from Nigeria (Dr. O. Ladipo), and there were three members from each of the world's developing regions. Funded by the Rockefeller Foundation, it was one of the most successful programs we funded during my years as director of Population Sciences. A meeting of South-to-South, hosted by the Indonesian member, Dr. Biran Affandi, was the purpose of the trip to Bali.

Ovulation suppression is the main mechanism of action of Norplant. During the first two years of use, 80–90% of cycles are clearly anovulatory (no eggs are released). By the fifth year, about 50% of cycles have blood hormone levels indicative of ovulation. Because the high level of contraceptive protection covers the entire five-year span, there must be another mechanism of action in addition to ovulation suppression. The secondary mechanism is the prevention of sperm from ascending into the female reproductive tract, so that fertilization cannot occur. This is achieved through an effect on the woman's cervical mucus. In a normal cycle, the mucus becomes less viscous and more abundant at about mid-cycle, facilitating sperm transport when ovulation is about to occur. In Norplant users, the mucus remains scanty, thick, and impenetrable to sperm.

As we studied Norplant, we understood that for some women, it is important, because of their religious or cultural beliefs, to know if interruption of early pregnancy plays a role in the mechanism of action. All available scientific methods have been applied to study this matter. They have been carried out in many independent laboratories, including the Catholic University in Santiago, Chile, where Dr. Horacio Croxatto was able to search for and recover human eggs at the end of a menstrual cycle to determine if they were fertilized. The Norplant studies include egg recovery, ovarian and uterine ultra-sound to detect ovulation or blastocyst formation, postcoital tests for sperm penetration, and efforts to detect the pregnancy hormone human chorionic gonadotropin (hCG) in the blood serum of women using Norplant. I participated in one of these studies in collaboration with Dr. Pentti Tuohima of Tampere, Finland, and Dr. Frank Alvarez of Santo Domingo, Dominican Republic. Pentti, who had been a postdoctoral fellow in my New York laboratory, had developed a new and ultra-sensitive test for hCG. When I read his scientific report that his new method could detect even trace amounts of the pregnancy hormone if it is present, I asked him to join us in the Norplant project. By all of these means it is clearly established that Norplant is a prefertilization method of contraception, even in cycles when ovulation has not been suppressed. It does not cause abortion or otherwise interfere with postfertilization events.

Shortly after the FDA announcement of Norplant's approval, the press and some legislators raised the issue of its potential use for "social engineering." Editorial writers were quick to suggest that women, particularly adolescents, receiving welfare payments from government might be tempted with incentives to accept a free Norplant insertion in order to avoid having more children. I was surprised when a conservative Republican congressman from Florida invited me for a breakfast discussion on how a federal program linking aid for dependent children and Norplant use might be structured. A state judge in California offered a woman convicted of child abuse the choice of Norplant or prison. After nearly 10 years of use elsewhere around the world without problems of this sort, these reproductive rights abuses started to surface within 10 days of its use in the United States.

As a scientist involved in the development of Norplant, I unequivocally and publicly opposed the coercive use of the method, or any other method of birth control, under any circumstances. I wrote letters to the *New York Times* and other newspapers expressing my opposition to the judge's action in California (which was ultimately dropped).

Janet Benshoof and her legal staff at the Center for Reproductive Rights, mostly young women, kept me informed about state legislatures considering bills that involved incentives or coercion as an inducement to use Norplant so that I could write a personal letter of opposition to each one. That wonderful group of public service lawyers works tirelessly to protect reproductive rights and freedom in the United States. Since the World Trade Center tragedy, homeland defense has been given high priority. The center's diligent efforts were a form of homeland defense long before the new cabinet-level post was created in Washington, D.C.

In spite of our efforts to protect against abuses, Norplant became the target of criticism by some feminist and consumer advocates opposed to a method that a woman could not control herself or might be coerced into using. These critics ignored the fact that implants can be removed at any time and fertility returns rapidly. And there was more trouble ahead.

Medical and scientific findings regarding the safety and effectiveness of Norplant have been affirmed and reaffirmed. Nevertheless, the method, like the IUD before it and most other contraceptives, soon became the target of product liability litigation in the United States. Although none of the claims have been upheld in courts around the country, the avalanche of adverse publicity caused a sharp drop in the use of Norplant. Women were coming into clinics with their lawyers, not their doctors, to ask for Norplant removals. A familiar question heard in women's clinics was, "Can you put them back in after I get my money?" What prompted this outbreak of litigation was the attempt on the part of trial lawyers to establish a class action against Wyeth-Ayerst, the product's distributor. Class action judgments can be extremely lucrative for lawyers, and some had just had a windfall in the Dow-Corning cases involving silicone-based breast implants. The new army of interested litigators was those who had taken their basic training on breast implant cases. When they heard about Norplant, they read "Silastic" and it sounded like a new gold strike.

Advertisements were placed in newspapers around the country, giving an 800 number with the enticing message that if you are using Norplant, we may be able to get you some money. By 1997, when 1 million American women were using Norplant, roughly 25,000 users signed up to be included in 200 law suits, 50 of which were attempts to get class action certification. Wyeth-Ayerst's lawyers, led by the brilliant young attorney, Robin Jacobsohn, were successful in defending Norplant in the courts of law around the country, but the negative publicity could not be erased, and the product's popularity plummeted.

Elsewhere the product has remained popular. By 2001, more than 10 million women had used it in the 60 countries where Norplant is registered. In the United States, the lawsuits have ended. To put an end to the large legal costs that were mounting, the defendant in the law suits, Wyeth-Ayerst, agreed in the summer of 1999 to a modest settlement per plaintiff, most of which probably went as fees for the plaintiffs' lawyers. Unfortunately, this has not stopped another law firm from yet another attempt to obtain class action certification; this is now working its way through the courts.

Norplant, in spite of its legal problems, paved the way for other long-acting contraceptive implants as several companies recognized the commercial potential of this new method. A number of new hormonal implant methods that require fewer implants than the six steroid-filled tubes of Norplant are now marketed or will be available in the near future. This reduction in number of implants is extremely important because it simplifies the implant insertion and removal.

Implanon is a single-rod system that is effective for three years. Developed by Organon of the Netherlands and marketed in Europe, it uses the same progestin, ketodesorgestrel, found in the company's popular oral contraceptive products. This is a third-generation super-progesterone which is even more potent that levonorgestrel. This is why the system can work with only a single implant. The company is ready to request FDA approval in the United States, but Organon may hold off on this for a while for corporate strategy purposes. They have another contraceptive innovation that they wish to introduce earlier, a vaginal contraceptive ring called Nuvaring.

When one of the research scientists at Organon was first promoting the idea within his company to use their super-progesterone for an implant, he invited me to Oss, the Netherlands, the company's headquarters, to give a presentation on implant contraception to Organon's high-level officials. I thought they had a winner because of their compound's high potency. Ketodesorgestrel seemed like a natural for implant technology, and I told them so. Later, they asked if we would jointly work with Organon on the product's development, but by then I was at the Rockefeller Foundation and it would not have been in keeping with foundation policy. I suggested that they work with the ICCR, but the two organizations could not agree on a contract. The company did an excellent job on their own, and I think their product will prove to be very successful. Instead of Silastic, which was going through its legal tribulations in the United States, they switched to another biocompatible polymer called ethylvinyl acetate and devised an excellent package which includes a preloaded inserter. Implanon is marketed in Europe and elsewhere and has been approved by the U.S. FDA.

Another new implant system, Jadelle, is marketed in Finland and has received FDA approval for marketing in the United States. The European Community countries in 2000 sanctioned its use as a five-year method. It consists of two flexible rods that release the same hormone used in Norplant and provides excellent protection against pregnancy for 5 years. Like Norplant, it rarely fails. The pregnancy rate is 0.2%, and its continuation-of-use rate is generally more than 80% per year. Jadelle started life as "Norplant II." Soon after starting clinical studies with the six-capsule system, we learned that the same blood levels of levonorgestrel could be achieved by using two, slightly longer flexible solid rods made by mixing the steroid with liquefied Silastic and then adding a polymerizing agent or fixative. Initially, doctors were reporting back that the rods had a tendency to break during the removal process. At a meeting on the problem, one of the laboratory technicians in New York suggested that we cover the rod with thin tubing. It was a good idea, and it worked after someone else in the lab figured out how to expand the tubing temporarily to get the rod inside.

After we had considerable data on this promising system, the U.S. Environmental Protection Agency labeled the fixative as potentially carcinogenic. Even though their concern pertained to doses 30,000 times as high as the amount in our implants, work had to stop until a way was found to replace the fixing agent with another approved material. The ultimate design of Jadelle became much more sophisticated than our original efforts with Silastic rods. It still has the thin-walled silicone tubing on the exterior.

Because it is FDA-approved, Jadelle could reach the U.S. market at any time as a three-year method. Its future is in the hands of Wyeth-Ayerst, at a time when the company is understandably gun-shy about product liability exposure. They spent more than $40 million defending Norplant before deciding in 2002 to discontinue the product. The amount of data assembled on the performance of Jadelle is enormous. It would be a loss to American women if the contraceptive system were not made available in the United States.

Other new implant methods still in the pipeline are single-implant systems that last one or two years. These are being developed in China, Brazil, and in the United States. If these products are brought to market, women will be able to select an implant system that provides one, two, three, or five years of near-perfect effectiveness, an important aid in achieving desired birth interval. This choice will include a system that can be used safely by mothers who are breast-feeding.

I referred to implant contraception as the first new methodology to be approved by the FDA in 30 years (when it won approval in 1991) because DepoProvera, a three-monthly injection of the progestin medroxyprogesterone acetate (DMPA), was not approved for use as a contraceptive in the United States until 1993, after having been used in more than 40 other countries for decades. It was first proposed as a contraceptive in 1966 when Coutinho reported that a dose of 150 milligrams DMPA administered intramuscularly causes temporary sterility by inhibiting ovulation for at least three months. It was another striking example of serendipity in research. As I mentioned earlier, Coutinho had been a postdoctoral student in the Rockefeller Institute laboratory of Dr. George Corner. When he returned to Brazil, he carried with him a small supply of a new progestin provided by the Upjohn Company of Kalamazoo, Michigan. His research specialty was uterine muscle activity, and the practical application of what he did was to try to prevent premature labor, a problem that is still difficult to manage. Following a then-current theory about the role of progesterone, Coutinho treated several of his patients with large doses of DMPA in order to save their pregnancies. Although the results for the original purpose were disappointing, he had the insight to realize that the treatment prevented ovulation for half a year. Coutinho undertook a series of studies involving women who did not wish to conceive and found that, depending on the dose, ovulation could be stopped for one, three, or six months. He published these results, but his originality tended to be overlooked by colleagues north of the equator. I not only knew about it, but had it in mind when I invited him to join the ICCR. Two years after the DMPA publication, he reported that conception control with less disturbance of menstrual bleeding can be achieved by monthly injections of DMPA combined with an estrogen.

After many years of neglect and quiescence, both the DepoProvera three-month injectable contraceptive and the combination-injectable product have been reintroduced in some countries, backed by extensive research sponsored by the World Health Organization. The World Health Organization's program on human reproduction started a research effort to find a new and improved injectable contraceptive. They used DMPA as the gold standard against which new candidates were tested. After several years of disappointments, someone had the bright idea, "Hey, why waste time and money looking for a new one when DMPA works just fine!" So, like an aging athlete, Depoprovera had a comeback, and its owner, Upjohn, took a renewed interest in its 40-year-old contestant in the contraceptive arena. The same revival of interest occurred with Coutinho's original combination-monthly injectable now marketed in several countries as Cyclofem and as Lunelle in the United States.

There will also be other delivery systems for contraceptive hormones. I have already described Mirena, the intrauterine system that releases a super-progesterone (levonorgestrel). The FDA announced its approval in December 2000 and its sponsor, Berlex Company (the American subsidiary of Schering, Berlin) began marketing in the United States in 2001 after successfully launching the contraceptive product in Europe.

Hormone-releasing vaginal rings have the advantage that a woman can control the method herself without the need for a clinic. One product, developed through the efforts of the World Health Organization's research program, was near commercial distribution when it fell victim to the problem I mentioned earlier, resulting from the withdrawal of the silicone plasticizer. Rather than start all over again with a new component, the interested company withdrew. There now is a fully studied combination-hormone vaginal ring developed by the ICCR; a company is needed to distribute it. It performs well both in terms of effectiveness and bleeding control, so it is likely to make it all the way to product introduction. This project has been of constant interest to Dr. Daniel Mishell, Jr., an ICCR founding member, and professor of obstetrics and gynecology at the University of Southern California. Meanwhile, Organon has developed its own vaginal ring which will be the first contraceptive of its kind on the market. The expected marketing strategy will delay the introduction of Implanon in the United States. Organon, with a relatively small operation in the United States, will launch the vaginal ring product first and hold off seeking approval for its implant contraceptive until a later date.

A contraceptive skin patch, Ortho Evra, that needs to be changed just once a week, was introduced in 2002 by Ortho-MacNeil Pharmaceuticals, and a second contraceptive patch is under development by the Agile Corporation of Wayne, Pennsylvania. Although these procedures, the ring and the patch, deliver the same hormones as oral contraceptives, they offer two advantages. They simplify the schedule of use; taking a pill every day is not easy for everyone. The hormones enter the bloodstream by absorption through the vaginal wall or the skin and therefore reach the general circulation without first passing through the liver. This is a pharmacological advantage for drug delivery.

The conventional combination pill is just as effective when used by placing it in into the vagina as it is when taken orally. A product approved, packaged, and marketed as a "vaginal pill" is being sold in Brazil after its effectiveness was established in a large international study. The positive results of the study were not unexpected because it had been shown in several clinical studies that contraceptive steroids can be absorbed through the vaginal wall. In fact, the levels of the pill's hormones in the blood are more consistent after vaginal absorption than after oral ingestion. Like the vaginal ring, the vaginal pill has the advantage of bypassing the liver when the drug first enters the bloodstream. Women who experience nausea or gastric upset when using an oral contraceptive can benefit from using the pill vaginally. The vaginal pill contraceptive, marketed by Biolab Sanus, a Brazilian company, is a success story of the South-to-South group mentioned earlier. All the data required for registration in Brazil were acquired from studies carried out by scientists in the developing world working cooperatively on this project. The product, named Lovelle, has become popular in Brazil and could be licensed by companies in other developing countries (as well as the United States, for that matter).

Postcoital contraception that could prevent a pregnancy from becoming established has been possible for several decades. Until recently, there has been no commercial interest in a product development effort, and few health care providers were aware of the effectiveness of "off-label" use of existing products for this purpose. Now, thanks to the efforts of several women's health advocacy groups, there is an emerging interest in what has come to be called "emergency contraception," and two dedicated products are sold in many countries, including the United States. Both eastern and western European countries have been far ahead of the United States in making these products available. I have been checking pharmacies in Switzerland, France, Germany, and Hungary during the past 10 years and could always find the products marketed by the Schering Company of Berlin, or the Hungarian Gideon-Richter Company. Both companies have been hesitant to do battle with the legal system and opponents of postfertilization contraception in the United States.

During the 1960s, orally active estrogenic products were shown to cause menstrual-like bleeding when taken within a few days of an unprotected intercourse. Bleeding and sloughing of the uterine lining means that pregnancy cannot take place even if a fertilized egg is present. I have already mentioned Hertig and Rock, the Boston doctors who studied fertilized human eggs. They found that normally about one-third to one-half of all fertilized eggs do not make it through the next expected menses because they are lost with the sloughed-off endometrium. Forty years ago the product used most frequently to cause this was diethylstilbestrol (DES). One study, done at a university student health service, found that no pregnancies occurred among 1000 young women who took DES within 6 days of unprotected intercourse, near mid-cycle. The main disadvantage was that the doses used caused severe nausea and vomiting. Other estrogens were tried but presented the same problem. This was an era when there was great caution over the use of estrogens, so that the few scientific papers that were published did little to elicit professional or commercial interest.

Subsequently, it was demonstrated that a high dose of the conventional pill, a combination of estrogen and progestin, can prevent pregnancy from becoming established when taken up to 72 hours after intercourse. This work prompted greater interest, and the method's use was adopted mainly by emergency room physicians treating rape victims and by student health services on university campuses. Companies marketing oral contraceptives in North America have been unwilling to label their products to indicate this activity, although the identical combination pill is the basis of the Schering product that can be found throughout Europe. In the United States the FDA responded to a petition, filed by the Center for Reproductive Rights (CRR), by convening a panel of experts who unanimously endorsed the conclusion that the method is safe and effective. However, the companies with appropriate products on the market continue to refuse to include this use in their labeling, even though this may be a violation of drug labeling laws, according to CRR's founding president, Janet Benshoof. The big companies have threatened to pull their oral contraceptive products off the market rather than label them as morning-after pills. This is reminiscent of the 1950s decision of Parke-Davis to deny that their original progestin was intended to be used as an oral contraceptive. In the present situation, I understand the pharmaceutical industry's anxiety about getting their oral contraceptives entangled in the abortion debate, but I can't see them walking away from a $2.5 billion market.

A small start-up, single-product company has sponsored a new drug application and now has its product on the market. It is called Prevens and consists of 4 high-dose oral contraceptive pills to be taken in 48 hours. It does not eliminate the nausea and vomiting problem I mentioned, but it is effective. This product includes a pregnancy test in the package, which increases the price considerably. Doctors have learned to break up the conventional oral contraceptive packages to get the same pills a lot cheaper.

The World Health Organization has sponsored studies of an anti-progesterone, mifepristone (discussed below), as an emergency contraceptive, with results that are extremely promising. Without an estrogenic component, the compound is equal in effectiveness to the high-dose combination pill method and causes far fewer of the transient side effects. The same is true of the second product I mentioned, marketed initially in Hungary. It is a progestin-only product now being duplicated by other companies, assuring wider distribution. It is distributed in the United States under the name PlanB. In an effort to disseminate information about emergency contraception, the population program of Princeton University started a hotline that women could call and get the name of the nearest doctor prepared to prescribe the needed product. The hotline had immediate success, receiving 1500 calls per week, and was expanded to include a web site. Even more amazing, I think, is the success of a similar program in Mexico City. Launched in February 1999, during the first year, the hotline was getting 3,000 calls a week, and the web site received 600,000 hits in a little over a year. The hotline was set up by the imaginative and dedicated women in the Population Council's Mexico City office. During the planning phase, my friend Gregorio Perez-Palacio, who headed the Ministry of Health's family planning services, urged me to talk them out of it, at least temporarily, because of problems he was having with the Catholic Church. I had to tell him that knowing Ana Langer and Charlotte Ellerton as I do, he could forget about it! The project became so huge a success that it has demonstrated the need and Perez-Palacio has asked Langer and Ellerton to expand the hotline to other cities in Mexico.

An adequate level of progesterone in a woman's blood is necessary for the establishment and maintenance of pregnancy. Compounds that do not act like progesterone but are able to occupy progesterone receptor sites on target cells (in the uterus, for example) prevent the natural hormone from carrying out its progestational role and are, therefore, contragestational. The first of these progesterone antagonists (the more accurate name is progesterone-receptor modifier) is mifepristone (RU-486), and by 1999 it had been registered as an approved drug for medical abortion in France, China, Sweden, and the United Kingdom and used successfully by more than one-half million women. In 2000 it was approved in the United States. It may have been in the nick of time for American women since an antiabortion administration and an increasingly antagonistic Supreme Court gradually chip away the rights supposedly assured under *Roe vs. Wade.* It is not at all certain that mifepristone will be exempted from the constraints being placed on access to abortion services, but it will be harder to regulate out of existence than conventional procedures to safely terminate early pregnancies.

Abortion induction has been the first clinical application of this important new class of drugs. The first studies used mifepristone alone. The success rate in women with established pregnancies who had missed their periods and were less than three weeks late ranged from 64 to 85%. The lack of response in some women was most likely due to inadequate uterine contractility. The combination of mifepristone with a prostaglandin (misoprostol), which induces contractions, given 48 hours later by intramuscular injection, by vaginal suppository, or taken orally, has resulted in a rate of complete abortion exceeding 90%. The oral route has become the therapy of choice. The combination is highly effective up to nine weeks since the last menstrual period.

Political opposition to mifepristone in the United States prevented its availability as a medical abortifacient for several years after it was introduced in Europe and has impeded progress on the investigation of its use for a number of other indications in gynecology and oncology. Unwilling to remain in the eye of the storm of controversy, the Roussel-UCLAF Company of Paris (now a part of the Hoechst Marion Roussel group) assigned all North American rights to mifepristone to the Population Council. Edouard Sakiz did not hold any grudges over his R2010 disappointment. An American clinical trial was completed, and the council submitted a new drug application for review by the FDA. The relevant advisory committee recommended approval and the FDA issued its approval in 2000, without restrictions that would have limited its availability. The council has transferred its rights to a commercial company so that manufacture and distribution could begin. It remains to be seen if the newly appointed FDA officials, the Congress, or the Executive Branch will be successful in limiting access as they have threatened to do.

Meanwhile, another abortion pill procedure is being used. Like mifepristone, this method also involves using an abortifacient drug (methotrexate) in combination with misoprostol. Methotrexate is a potent antimetabolite that has a long history of use as a chemotherapeutic agent for the treatment of the embryonal cancer called choriocarcinoma. Methotrexate interferes with cell division by acting as an inhibitor of folic acid. In recent years, at lower doses than those used for cancer therapy, the drug has been used for the nonsurgical treatment of some ectopic pregnancies and at even lower doses for alleviating the symptoms of arthritis and some dermatologic disorders. Now the abortifacient use, first suggested more than 30 years ago, is being reconsidered and is currently under investigation with FDA authorization.

The main advantage of methotrexate–misoprostol would be that the two drugs are already approved and in use for other purposes. They could, therefore, be prescribed for an off-label use without additional FDA authorization. The main disadvantage from a user's perspective is the prolonged time required to initiate and complete a medical abortion by this procedure. Doctors may be reluctant to prescribe a potent antimetabolite for an off-label purpose that might be difficult to defend in the event of malpractice litigation.

Using human chorionic gonadotropin (hCG) as the antibody-stimulating component is the best chance of developing a contraceptive vaccine. The rationale is to develop antibodies that will interfere with the establishment and maintenance of an early pregnancy. If hCG is neutralized by antibodies at the time of the next expected menses, endometrial sloughing and a menstrual flow would occur whether or not a fertilized egg is present. The most advanced approach uses the principle of coupling a component of the native hCG molecule to a carrier protein to create a more potent and effective vaccine. The carrier protein is usually tetanus toxoid or diphtheria toxin, substances that have proven to be relatively safe as vaccines in large-scale use in human populations. Work done primarily in India uses a synthetic molecule that resembles the three-dimensional shape of hCG. Pran Talwar is the leader of this work.

The Indian vaccine induces a temporary immunization of short duration so that frequent booster shots are required to maintain antibody levels above the threshold required for effective hCG neutralization. This feature is sometimes overlooked by critics who are concerned about the potential irreversibility of an hCG vaccine. The development of adjuvants that would permit a feasible and acceptable schedule for reversibility, but with longer periods of immunization, is necessary.

Research on the development of contraceptive vaccines has become controversial. Some women's health advocates have expressed grave concern about the potential for misuse of an antifertility vaccine. They fear its involuntary or coerced application to sterilize women forcibly. Given this perceived potential for abuse, they question the ethics of working on contraceptive vaccines and call for restraint on the part of scientists and organizations that support scientific research. At least one start-up biotechnology company that initially undertook a development program for an anti-hCG vaccine has discontinued its investment in the face of this opposition.

None of the contraceptive advances I have written about offer a woman protection against sexually transmitted diseases, including HIV/AIDS. This is a supremely important issue in AIDS-affected countries around the world. Now, the most seriously threatened regions are central, eastern, and southern Africa. An estimated 20% of young adults in South Africa are HIV positive. Most will die because there is no practical treatment that can reach them in time. Thailand, India, and Nepal have high incidences of HIV positivity. Because of its large population, the absolute toll of AIDS in Asia could exceed that of Africa. The independent states of the former Soviet Union are also experiencing a serious epidemic.

Our tools to combat this terrible pandemic are condom use and behavior modification. We need to find methods that women can use to protect themselves from sexually transmitted diseases, including HIV. Women throughout the world are confronted with the growing risk of infection with HIV. Consistent condom use is not always feasible for many women, since it requires male approval and participation. The vaginal sheath, vaginal virucidal creams or gels, medicated condoms, or other means to reduce infection of women are urgently needed. This is a complicated line of research that cannot depend on laboratory results alone. Ultimately, clinical trials will be required, and the design of such trials presents daunting challenges. Some explorations are in progress, but this research should receive a much higher allocation of resources and the attention of scientists, commercial companies, and funding agencies throughout the world.

There is no ideal contraceptive method that will meet all the needs of the world's diverse population. Although the advances beyond the pill and IUD have been numerous, we cannot be complacent about contraceptive technology. How can we when, in spite of the methods now available, half of the unplanned and unwanted pregnancies in the United States occur because of contraceptive failure? How do we explain that we cannot offer methods that are both effective and offer protection against sexually transmitted diseases? And how do we rationalize that the world still has a large unmet need for contraceptive services? In part, this is due to the barriers that have been erected to impede contraceptive distribution and development, but we must acknowledge that something is lacking in our array of technology.

I mentioned earlier that the three-year period from 2000 through 2002 will bring a record number of launches of new contraceptive products. Mirena, Implanon, Ortho Evra, Nuvaring, Lunelle, Jadelle, and PlanB are some of the products that have appeared. They introduce new methods of contraception using implants, patches, vaginal rings, intrauterine systems, or morning-after pills. Yet, scientists who follow us at the next turn of century will probably look back at these early years of the twenty-first century and think we were quaint or even primitive with our technologies. They may marvel at how we were able to get along with our limited understand of biological processes. To believe otherwise would be the height of scientific hubris.

6

Is Contraceptive Research a Male Chauvinist Plot?

When I lecture on advances in contraception, I'm sometimes asked by a woman in the audience, "What about contraceptives for men?" The implication of the question, sometimes not only implied but bluntly asserted, is that contraceptive research is done by male researchers, funded by agencies controlled by men, and, consciously or inadvertently, protects the male by seeking methods that place the responsibility and risk on women.

It is absolutely true that contraceptive innovations of recent decades have been methods that are used by women. This would have delighted Margaret Sanger, the early fighter for women's reproductive rights, who inspired the search for a contraceptive pill for women. Her fight against the repressive Comstock laws that made disseminating contraception information or materials illegal was a struggle for this principle. She faced and accepted imprisonment for demanding that women be given control of their own reproduction. Yet, some modern feminists see the emphasis on contraceptive methods for women as a male chauvinist plot.

The Cairo agenda calls for contraception research based on a "woman-centered agenda" that includes contraceptive methods for males that would both expand the range of contraceptive choice and their sharing in the responsibility for contraception. It is also the message of Cairo that men should be encouraged and enabled to take responsibility for their sexual and reproductive behavior. The dominant message of Cairo on contraception, however, is that women should control contraceptive methods used and that they should not be under the control of a male partner.

The bewildering part of the feminist demand for more male contraceptives is that when couples use contraception that depends on the active participation of men, women tend to have accidental pregnancies more often than when female-controlled methods are used. Perhaps this is the reason that more and better male methods are needed. Or perhaps it reflects the unreliability of men when it comes to using contraception. If he doesn't get it right, it is the woman who pays the price. You've heard it said: There would be fewer accidents if it were the man who gets pregnant!

It is a simple matter to estimate the number of unplanned pregnancies that will occur each year as a result of contraceptive failure. Based on the number of users of methods in the United States and known failure rates of those methods, it can be calculated that nearly 1 million of the 1.6 million contraceptive failure pregnancies that occur each year are among users of condoms, withdrawal, and rhythm (which requires male partner cooperation). What this means is that although less than 20% of contraceptive use requires male participation, these methods result in well over half of all contraceptive failures in the United States.

The global perspective adds to the bewilderment. Surveys have been done in Africa and Asia concerning husband's attitudes toward fertility, contraceptive use, and reproductive preferences. Compared to their wives, men want more children, not fewer. In the west African countries in the survey, the ideal family size reported by men was nine, well above the upper limit preferred by women. Up to 90% of men claimed they wanted more children, regardless of how many they had at the time of the survey. On the brighter side, compared to married women, men generally report higher levels of knowledge about contraceptive methods and just a slightly lower approval rate of family planning compared to women.

This makes a shaky case for diverting funds from other purposes to support male contraceptive research. I cannot believe that women's health advocates and feminist leaders are demanding more research on male contraception so that more of the responsibility for women's reproductive health will depend on men. No doubt there is a need to involve men in reproduction decisions, but to do so at the cost of women giving up control in the vital matter of contraceptive use is a questionable trade-off.

I believe the underlying rationale for demanding greater attention to male methods is so men can share with women the perceived health risks of contraception. This justification fails to recognize that the perceived risk of modern contraceptives far exceeds the real risk. By 1987 there was ample medical and scientific evidence to document the safety of both oral contraceptives and IUDs. Yet, an analysis that year of attitudes regarding risk behavior published in *Science* magazine showed that oral contraceptives were perceived by the public to be high up on the scale of risky activities. Perceived risk is based on media reports and anecdotal stories. Real risk is based on evidence and scientifically grounded conclusions.

In mid 2002 the press carried accounts of an article in the *Journal of the American Medical Association* that was abruptly halted because, it was reported, the unexpected risks of hormone replacement therapy (HRT) for women were greater than the benefits. The facts were different. Parts of the study continue as planned. The arm that was discontinued was stopped according to a pre-planned formula. Important benefits for taking HRT were not included in establishing this early ending plan. Anxious women started phoning their doctors, some dangerously abandoned their medication, editorials were written, stock prices fell, and litigation lawyers started advertising for clients. Yet, the report merely confirmed that HRT causes a slight increase in diagnosed breast cancer without increasing mortality, and added data to the growing realization that HRT does not provide protection against heart disease, even though it changes the blood cholesterol profile in a heart-firendly direction. In simple terms the report found that if 100 women use HRT for five years, one of them would experience a non-fatal adverse event attributable to the use of the medication. This episode is a classical example of how perceived risk is generated.

In contraception research, perceived risk has had an important impact on policy and in the budget allocations of organizations that support contraceptive development. Several of these funding agencies have responded to the call for male contraceptive research in the context of a "women-centered agenda" by earmarking funds for this type of research.

Continuing research toward the development of new methods of contraception that would be used by men is both warranted and promising. In my laboratory we have worked on the possibility of a male vaccine, a male implant system, a reversible vasectomy, and a male pill. As a founding member of the International Society of Andrology, I have tried to encourage scientists to work in this field. What baffles me is why anyone would think that undertaking research on methods that would improve the options for women, under their own control, would be less valuable. No, I don't think that contraception research is a male chauvinist plot.

The lay press, fascinated by this subject, writes as much nonsense about contraceptives for men as they do about topics like miracle diets or secrets to living to 100. Not long ago, a Reuters story carried the headline "Mice hold clue to male contraceptive pill." It describes excellent work on a gene that produces a receptor protein in the muscle cells of the vas deferens of white mice. Knockout mice (mice bred without this gene) were less successful than normal male mice in inseminating females. From there to a male contraceptive pill is an amazing stretch of scientific credibility. My voice mail carries a message almost every week from a journalist seeking a comment about yet another new male contraceptive.

The most extensive clinical experience with a new male contraceptive has been accumulated with a pill tested mostly in China but also investigated in other countries. It consists of gossypol, the pigment that gives cottonseed a yellowish color. (The Latin name for the many varieties of cotton plants is *Gossypium*.) Among its other properties, gossypol endows the growing crop with protection against insects. Botanists and food chemists have been interested in gossypol for a long time. The reason for this interest was the prospect of using the cotton plant to produce gossypol-free cottonmeal as fodder for farm animals because the normal gossypol level can be toxic to certain farm animals. There is, in fact, a small industry in Israel that produces gossypol-free cottonmeal by chemical extraction. Plant breeders have been able to breed cotton plants with low gossypol content, but these varieties prove to be vulnerable to pest attack and do not survive in open fields.

The idea that gossypol could be used as a contraceptive in men sprung from the serendipitous observation that uncooked cottonseed oil (which contains gossypol) had been responsible for an epidemic of infertility in a rural area in China. The gossypol story in China unfolded during the Cultural Revolution when Chinese farmers were suffering a food shortage. Cottonseed oil is a staple in Chinese food preparation and is usually prepared by lengthy boiling of cottonseeds so that the protein content is precipitated out and the valuable cooking oil can be recovered. This process removes virtually all of the gossypol. To reduce the loss of oil in the cooking process, and to save on valuable firewood, some villages adopted a cold-press procedure to extract cottonseed oil, but this method does not remove the gossypol. No one suspected a problem until it was realized that there were no children being born in entire villages. Of course, the women were thought to be responsible, so when help was sought, gynecology experts were consulted.

A young woman doctor who had been ordered out into the countryside was in one of the villages, and she quickly came to the conclusion that it was an unknown environmental factor, or something in the food. She called upon professors at Peking Union Medical College in Beijing to help. An excellent pharmacologist, Dr. Lei Hai Peng, was part of the team sent to investigate, and so was the urologist Dr. Liu Guo Chen. By some marvelous medical sleuthing, these scientists pinned the cause for the infertility on the men and traced it back to gossypol. The important piece in the puzzle was Peng remembering a 1933 paper published in a Chinese traditional medicine journal in which the author mentioned male infertility in connection with the therapeutic use of gossypol. Apparently, the substance has had a long history of use in traditional medicine for various illnesses.

Another important clue was that the one woman who conceived in a particular village was married to a soldier in the People's Liberation Army, who came back to be with her only for a short time during his leave of absence. The investigation prompted the Chinese Academy of Medical Sciences to establish a nationwide coordinating group on male infertility agents. By 1978 the group published a report of its study on gossypol as an antifertility agent for men.

For some reason, the Chinese chose to be secretive about this work. I suspect it was because of the episode's connection with the austere living conditions during the Cultural Revolution. As a guest of the Chinese Academy of Sciences, I visited China in both 1977 and 1978 to lecture around the country on contraceptive research, and this project was never mentioned to me. I picked up some signals that there was something going on, but I could never pin it down. It's too bad because I think I could have offered some suggestions that would have improved the value of their work.

More than 10,000 Chinese men were enrolled in studies using several doses of gossypol. The initial countrywide project reported a success rate of 99.4% for suppressing sperm production to levels believed to be incompatible with fertility. The report selected cases that began taking a daily 20-milligram pill for approximately 3 months and then reduced use to a pill every other day. The antifertility effect was achieved without lowering testosterone levels in blood so that, unlike other approaches to male contraception, add-back hormone replacement therapy to maintain libido and other secondary sexual characteristics was not required. For me, that was the eye-catching aspect of the gossypol report: the ability to stop sperm production without stopping male hormone production. This problem had been an obstacle in many other approaches to male contraception.

By any standards of clinical research, there were serious problems with the design of the Chinese study. Each center used its own source of gossypol so that the medication used was not standardized. Various doses were used, and other differences made it questionable for the results from each center to be combined. Nevertheless, in the final report, reduction in blood potassium levels (hypokalemia) was flagged as an issue of concern, particular by officials at the Contraceptive Development Branch of the U.S. National Institute of Child Health and Human Development and the World Health Organization, and this matter has clouded subsequent attitudes toward the potential use of gossypol as a male contraceptive.

Without adequate controls, it was not possible to gauge the association of gossypol to this change in blood chemistry. Although several scientists have attempted to establish an animal model or a mechanism of action for this imputed effect of gossypol, results have not been definitive. Subsequently, when gossypol has been tested as a contraceptive in countries other than China, no evidence of potassium loss has been reported. An international comparative study determined that plasma potassium levels of Chinese men tend to be lower than the values of men in other countries and that this appears to be related to dietary rather than to genetic factors. Designed and supervised by Dr.

Marcus Reidenberg, director of the Division of Clinical Pharmacology of Cornell Medical School in New York, an international study was even able to demonstrate that men from Shanghai living in the United States have higher potassium blood levels that the average in Shanghai. This was another of the successful projects of South-to-South, mentioned earlier.

Another problem that confuses the study of safety issues is the large difference in daily dose to stop sperm production in men compared to laboratory animals. Sperm production in men can be stopped with 1/200 or less than the dose required in monkeys, rats, rabbits, or mice. This means that, on a body-weight basis, men need much lower doses than those used in typical animal studies that have been done.

The issue of toxicity influenced the World Health Organization's involvement in gossypol research. Shortly before the Chinese announcement, the World Health Organization had decided to terminate efforts to develop a male contraceptive, using the rationale that no promising leads were available. With the publicity of the Chinese work and the prodding of India's Prime Minister Indira Gandhi, the decision was reconsidered. The World Health Organization program collaborated with Chinese scientists to learn about what happened to the men who had taken gossypol during the Chinese trials and gathered information of animal toxicity which they believed supported the earlier decision not to support new studies on gossypol. The World Health Organization did invest in work to modify gossypol and underwrote a costly animal toxicity study. After deciding that gossypol would not be acceptable as an antifertility drug, the World Health Organization turned its attention to another herbal extract taken from Chinese traditional medicine, *Tripterygium wilfordii*, derived from a root found in southern China. This work is continuing.

After the report in the *China Medical Journal*, I accompanied a team to China, sponsored by the Rockefeller Foundation, to learn more about the work with gossypol. Chinese doctors who had participated in the studies organized a fact-finding mission. We were invited to China by the Chinese Academy of Medical Sciences. I took the team's advice to support the Chinese efforts and learn more about the potential of gossypol as a male contraceptive. After all, the team members pointed out, gossypol had been used in Chinese traditional medicine for hundreds of years. Dr. Liu Guo Chen, the urologist involved in the identification of gossypol-induced male infertility, claimed that, over the years, more Chinese people using traditional medicine had taken gossypol than Westerners had ever used aspirin. In a country with a population of more than 1 billion, it's a believable assertion. In our visits to several of the centers where the Chinese work on male contraception had been done, it was evident that there was a difference of opinion among the Chinese doctors.

I was particularly impressed with Liu. He taught me about life in China from the Great Leap Forward in the 1950s through the Cultural Revolution and all the other social upheavals in between. I asked him how he was able to endure the great shifts that influenced everyone's personal and family life. "Life is like sailing a boat, Dr. Segal," he answered, "You go where the wind takes you and look for a safe harbor when the winds are too strong." In Beijing, Liu took me on a tour of the Peking Union Medical College (PUMC), China's premier medical school, which had been created by the Rockefeller Foundation's philanthropy in 1917. I was the first Rockefeller Foundation officer to receive permission from higher authorities to make a post-Revolution visit to PUMC, so this was a special occasion. As we toured the beautiful campus with its pagoda-style buildings, I told Liu that a friend of mine, James Grant, the late, revered head of UNICEF, had been born in that hospital. His father John Grant was a Rockefeller Foundation doctor working in China in the 1920s. "Jimmy Grant," he reflected softly. "He was in my Boy Scout troop." Life does, indeed, take some unpredictable tacks, as Dr. Liu knew only too well.

That visit to China was marked by the opportunity to host a reception for PUMC graduates who were given permission to assemble from all over China. It was a moving experience as they greeted me, astonished to realize that the Rockefeller Foundation still honored its ties to them.

With Liu's guidance, we undertook several studies on effectiveness, safety, and reversibility of gossypol as a male pill. First, we attempted to confirm the work at the dose the Chinese doctors had reported. No adverse reactions were noted, and the effectiveness was confirmed. Next, we did studies with a reduced dose following the pharmacological principle of seeking the minimal effective dose. In 2000, we were able to publish a scientific article describing the results of a study involving more than 150 men from Brazil, Nigeria, and Kenya (another South-to-South study.) The doses used were lower than those in the original Chinese study, and about 1/6 the dose Chinese doctors use for the treatment of some gynecological diseases. Our study appears to have used a dose that was just about on the borderline of effectiveness. Sperm production was stopped in 60% of the treated men. Although the dose used was not sufficiently effective to be practical, half of the men that did respond failed to resume sperm production a year after treatment ended. Otherwise, there were no side effects attributable to the drug. If gossypol is to be moved forward as a male contraceptive, more work will be needed to establish the proper dose, or chemical variations of the original molecule will have to evolve, improving performance with respect to both effectiveness and reversibility.

From what we now know, gossypol could have application as a medical alternative for men who do not require a guaranteed reversible method: a medical alternative to vasectomy. A Brazilian company that specializes in the development of pharmaceuticals from natural products, Hebron S/A of Pernambuco, has succeeded in extracting and purifying gossypol from Brazilian cotton plants on a large scale.

Another possible use of gossypol may pave the way to its entry on the market. Scientists in the Helsinki laboratory of one of the original ICCR members found that gossypol can prevent the replication of viruses that have a protein coat, but not naked DNA viruses. The specificity of this action prompted me to organize a study of gossypol's effect on the HIV virus. With the cooperation of Dr. Bruce Polsky, the laboratory work was done at Sloan-Kettering Cancer Research Institute in New York. The results showed that the enzyme responsible for HIV replication, reverse transcriptase, was inhibited in the presence of adequate concentrations of gossypol.

The facts were that gossypol reaches the testis and epididymis because it can stop sperm production in the testis and prevent motility from developing in sperm stored in the epididymis. The concentration of gossypol needed to achieve these effects can be reached if men take 20-milligram tablets once a day. As for safety of this dose, Chinese gynecologists routinely treat endometriosis with 40 milligrams daily for several months. Gossypol at an adequate concentration can prevent the replication of HIV in vitro. The question was, is the concentration found in the male reproductive tract adequate to prevent virus replication in semen? Another question was, where exactly is HIV in the semen? There are three possible compartments: there could be virus particles free in the seminal fluid; the virus could be located in infected white blood cells that are routinely found in semen; or it could be on the sperm.

The last possibility was a controversial matter, with some scientists claiming they could prove the presence of HIV on sperm by electron micrographs and others interpreting the micrographs differently. I tended to side with the nay-sayers on this issue but that didn't really matter for our hypothesis. If gossypol could work in vivo the same as it does in vitro, we should be able to eliminate the virus from the semen, even if it would not be a treatment for the underlying disease throughout the body. Our rationale was that the purpose of recommending safer sex (condom use) is to prevent the virus from being transmitted to a sexual partner. If this could also be achieved by a medicine, it would be useful in slowing the spread of AIDS.

A visiting oncologist at Sloan-Kettering, Dr. Mario Paredes, learned about our in vitro work and volunteered to undertake a small clinical trial with HIV patients in Guadalajara, Mexico. After receiving the necessary permission from authorities, he started treating a group of volunteer gay men who were HIV positive but had no other medication available to them. No one, in other words, would be deprived of other forms of treatment then available in Mexico.

After the study was running for several months, Polsky and I went down to Guadalajara for a review of progress. Paredes was able to confirm in these HIV-positive men the suppressing effect of gossypol on sperm production without influencing blood potassium levels. Paredes also observed that, over time, white blood cells disappeared from the semen samples of treated men. Usually, a semen analysis will disclose a certain number of white blood cells because almost all men have some slight degree of prostatitis or other asymptomatic reproductive tract infection.

During the day, we interviewed several of the patients who came in for their monthly checkups. That evening, when we boarded a plane for Mexico City, I recognized one of these men in the boarding lounge, and we sat together for the trip. He told me that he came from Mexico City at his own expense each month, taking a day off from his work as a bank clerk because it gave him a sense of purpose. He had not been misled and understood that there was no evidence that the gossypol treatment would benefit him in his fight against the dreaded disease, but he felt a fulfillment in participating in work that might, someday, help someone else, or prevent someone from being infected. I don't know the outcome of that man's personal history, but I hope his disease remained asymptomatic long enough for him to benefit from the anti-retroviral treatments that came along soon afterward. As for Paredes' work, it was sufficiently successful to prompt a follow-up study at Mexico's prestigious Institute of Nutrition in the capital city and that study also proved that the viral load in the semen of gossypol-treated men can be suppressed. This work serves as the basis for the Hebron Company's application to register gossypol for this purpose for mar-keting in Brazil.

In contrast to the serendipitous disclosure of gossypol's contracep-tive action in rural China, the discovery of gonadotropin-releasing hor-mone (GnRH) the small molecule from the brain that indirectly con-trols the function of the human gonads, was the product of sophisticated biotechnology that earned Nobel Prizes for two American scientists. After many years of research to utilize this discovery for contraception, the synthesis of antagonists of GnRH, free of undesir-able side effects, is a positive step toward a male contraceptive based on the principle of GnRH inhibition.

Gonadotropin-releasing hormone is a peptide that is digested if taken by mouth, so it is not active orally. Developing some other de-livery form that would be useful for contraception has been a challenge. Unlike the extensive experience with release of steroids from Silastic (Norplant) for long-acting delivery systems, there is no similar tech-nology to borrow from to create a delayed-release system for water-soluble peptides. To be practical, several criteria must be met. The de-livery system must use materials that can be used clinically without causing a local or systemic foreign-body reaction. Solubility and sta-bility of the peptide must be sufficient to permit storage of an adequate amount to assure a significant period of effectiveness. Release rate of the peptide from the vehicle must be slow and constant enough to provide a reasonably constant blood level over the period of use. Syn-thetic polymers similar to the one used for soft contact lens products may meet these requirements. Hydron, the plastic used in contact lenses, rarely initiates a foreign body reaction.

A male contraceptive method based on GnRH will need to meet another requirement. Because the releasing hormone indirectly controls both the sperm-producing and the hormone-producing functions of the testis, men treated with an antagonist to suppress sperm production would require androgen replacement therapy to maintain libido, potency, and other secondary male sex characteristics. Some form of testosterone would be required because this male hormone is involved in many biological functions besides libido and potency; it also regulates growth and function of muscle, kidney, liver, and bone. The development of suitable hormone replacement therapy for men is complicated by the fact that concurrent testosterone treatment can offset the inhibitory effect of GnRH analogues on sperm production.

Potential toxicity and metabolic issues further complicate the development of appropriate androgen replacement therapy. Unlike estrogens and progestins, most androgens currently available are not active when taken orally. When testosterone therapy is used for the treatment of sexual dysfunction or hypogonadism, frequent intramuscular injections are required. This can lead to wide fluctuations in concentrations in the blood over the effective time period of the injection. Although testosterone delivery systems such as pellets or microspheres that would last for six months may be feasible, they do not overcome all the shortcomings. Other delivery systems such as patches that are placed on the scrotum are also available. These, too, have their limitations.

Longer-acting super-androgens hold greater promise for a suitable sustained release form for androgen replacement therapy. One analogue of testosterone can be prepared in a polymeric matrix that has a life span of at least one year when placed subdermally. Used in conjunction with a GnRH analogue-releasing Hydron implant, this product could resolve many of the problems that have confronted researchers striving to develop a practical male contraceptive over the past several decades. In fact, this testosterone derivative, MENT, is sufficiently powerful as a gonadotropin inhibitor and weak as a prostate stimulator that its use alone for contraception seems very promising.

When we gave up on developing a male implant because testosteronelike compounds with adequate potency were not available, I could not have known that years later, the ICCR would ultimately come up with a solution. A talented biochemist, the late Carl Monder, working in the Population Council laboratories at the Rockefeller University, studied the biological activity of an unusual testosterone analogue that had been on the shelf for many years without getting much attention. Its chemical structure gives it the abbreviation MENT. He found that it is a super-androgen and that in the body it is not converted to the form of testosterone, called dihydrotestosterone or DHT, that stimulates the prostate and causes acne and balding. This advantage and other characteristics made it a perfect candidate for a male implant for hormone replacement therapy and for contraception. Teaming up with another Population Council scientist, Kalyan Sundaram, an impressive array of studies were carried out firmly establishing that MENT is not converted to DHT and that it is able to maintain the body's need for androgenic and anabolic (muscle-building) activity, usually the responsibility of testosterone.

Years of work have proved the safety of MENT and shown that subdermal implants can last for six months to a year. It can also be administered by skin patch or gel. Schering AG of Berlin has been licensed by the Population Council to develop some of these potential products. Like other androgenic and anabolic steroids, MENT will need to be monitored for misuse, particularly among athletes who may use these compounds to improve performance.

Although reports continue to surface from time to time on the use of injections of conventional androgens, progestins, or androgen-progestin combinations for the prevention of sperm production, it is unlikely that these research activities will lead to the development of an acceptable and practical system for male contraception. It has been nearly 40 years since steroidal suppression of gonadotropins was proposed as an approach to male contraception, and some of the same basic uncertainties remain today. Remember my story about the scary airplane ride back from my mid-winter visit to Detroit? The purpose of that trip was to discuss with Parke-Davis scientists the results my chief, Warren Nelson, had achieved in suppressing sperm production in rats by injections of their super-progesterone, norethindrone. Since the airlines were using the DC6 then, you can assume the idea has been around a long time.

Any method that risks exceeding physiological blood levels of testosterone would be viewed with skepticism because of the critical role of androgens in cardiovascular events, prostate stimulation, and other bodily functions. Careful monitoring would be required to prevent steroid abuse that has caused such compounds to be banned by the National Collegiate Athletic Association, the National Football League, the U.S. Olympic Committee, and the International Olympic Committee. It is hard to visualize the acceptability of a contraceptive product based on the use of the same hormones that disqualify athletes from competition. One need only observe the controversy aroused by the suggested approval of occasional medical use of marijuana to predict the outcry that would greet the suggested contraceptive use of a controlled substance like testosterone or its analogues.

Other compounds that have primary effects elsewhere in the body may also cause some degree of male infertility, which could be utilized for male contraception. Mifepristone (RU486) is one of these. It acts on the sperm's membrane, interfering with the ability of the sperm to take up calcium. Lacking calcium, sperm do not attain motility, and if they cannot move, they cannot fertilize the egg. The overall endocrine profile of mifepristone, however, would make it unacceptable for use in men. Mifepristone could, however, serve as a model for the synthesis of other compounds that would be more specific in their action. The same is true of a prescription drug, nifedipine, a calcium channel blocker that is used to reduce blood pressure. Dr. Susan Benoff of New York University believes that it causes sterility in men by preventing the final stage of sperm maturation. She claims that the drug prevents the sperm from releasing the enzymes that it needs to cut through the external coats to reach the egg's surface. There is no chance that this blood pressure-reducing drug will ever be used as a male contraceptive, but if its action is confirmed and could be found in other compounds that would not have general effects in the body, it would be an excellent mechanism because of its specificity.

Scientists are now exploring immunological means to suppress male fertility. One line of research is based on the principle of GnRH inhibition, similar to the use of antagonist analogues mentioned earlier. The GnRH molecule is too small to be significantly antigenic, but linking it to a carrier protein enhances its ability to stimulate antibody formation. With a vaccine based on this principle, GnRH-neutralizing antibodies would inhibit spermatogenesis, and androgen replacement therapy would ensure normal male secondary sex characteristics and functions. In another South-to-South project led by Pran Talwar, some men with prostate cancer have been immunized safely with a GnRH vaccine to suppress androgen stimulation of prostatic tissue. But these preliminary studies have not dealt with the issue of androgen replacement, an essential component of a vaccine that would be used to control fertility in normal men.

The potential availability of MENT implants brightens the chances for this type of vaccine, considerably. Vaccines are also envisaged that could prevent sperm maturation in the epididymis or prevent the passage of the sperm through the outer layers of the egg. Another would block fertilization by attaching antibodies to the protein sperm use as a landing gear on the egg's surface.

Technology, in itself, will not encourage the positive involvement of men as supportive partners in reproductive health. This will take education, the building of comfort and capacity to discuss contraception, and the willingness to come to joint decisions on a matter so personal in the lives of husband and wife. While bench scientists and doctors are working on their leads for male contraception, social scientists and community leaders must be making progress in changing the role and attitudes of men. This, too, was part of the challenge in the Cairo agenda.

7

Barriers to Developing New Contraceptives

People who wish to limit their fertility do so primarily in pursuit of family or individual aspirations. They want to enhance their chances for personal fulfillment and to provide a good home and opportunities for their children. The availability of effective contraceptive methods gives couples the opportunity to determine, with dignity and personal freedom, how many children they will have and when they will have them. This reproductive freedom is a human right, not a privilege reserved for the well-to-do. If because of inadequate education, poverty, or lack of health services, people do not have access to effective contraception, there is a de facto denial of this right. Families that are already struggling to meet the needs of existing children should not be deprived of the contraceptive services available to those who are better off. For the poorest of the poor, this struggle is often a matter of providing their children with adequate food and shelter.

Although there is still a large unmet need for contraception and millions continue to be frustrated by high rates of unwanted pregnancy, contraceptive use around the world has grown over the past 40 years. The number of couples using contraception or sterilization has increased more than tenfold. In the poorer countries, the number of contraceptive users has increased from under 50 million before 1960 to more than 600 million in 2000. The contraceptive prevalence rate has moved up from 8% to greater than 50% and is continuing to rise in most of the developing world. In the United States and other industrialized countries, the percentage of married couples using contraceptives (that's the way the U.S. Census Bureau reports the information) is in the 70–90% range.

With rising contraceptive use, fertility has been steadily declining. In developing countries, the number of children a woman will have in her lifetime has decreased from more than six in the 1960s to fewer than four, more than half way to the replacement level. China is already at replacement level, and India is moving toward that lower rate of fertility. India's overall contraceptive prevalence has climbed in recent years to more than 40% of couples in the reproductive age group, and the total fertility rate has fallen to 3.3. Most industrialized countries have fertility levels that barely replace existing population; many are even below replacement.

National surveys have provided detailed information on the methods that people choose. Surgical sterilization by tubal ligation ranks first among methods chosen by American couples. The pill is the most frequently used reversible method. In other countries the pattern is different. In China, Sweden, and France, the intrauterine device (IUD) is the preferred reversible method. Until 1999, modern hormonal methods for women were not available in Japan. The predominant method used is the condom. In actual practice, what this means is that men use the condom and women have uncomplicated access to legal and safe abortion when faced with a contraceptive failure.

Although the contraceptives that people choose differ from country to country or from culture to culture, methods that women use predominate. In Latin America and Africa, male use of contraception is negligible. In India surgical sterilization is the main method used to prevent pregnancy. There was a period some years ago when vasectomy was emphasized in the national family planning program in India, but currently, most sterilization operations are tubal ligations.

The distinguished Indian gynecologist, V. N. Shirodker (he developed an operation that is used throughout the world) tells the story of a wealthy mill owner from Bombay who came for a consultation in the days when tubal ligation was done by open abdominal surgery.

"I understand, Professor, that there's a way for my wife to stop having babies. We have three sons and that is sufficient."

"Yes," Shirodker replied. "Your wife will have to be admitted to my hospital . . . she will have general anesthesia for the surgery and she will be able to go home after a few days."

"General anesthesia? Surgery? Oh no, I love my wife very much and would not want to submit her to such a risk!"

Shirodkar reflected for a moment and said, "Well, there's a much simpler and faster operation that can be done here in the office with a local anesthetic."

"The safer one! That's what I want!," the mill owner exclaimed. "When should I bring her in!"

"No, you misunderstand," explained Dr. Shirodkar. "This procedure is done on you, not your wife. But it will have the same result in the end."

The loving husband thought this over and replied, "On second thought, the first method will be fine. I know you're an excellent surgeon and will take good care of my wife."

There are more vasectomies done in China than in all of the rest of the world combined. Some provinces of China rely heavily on vasectomy, so that in the country at large, men account for about 10% of contraceptive users. Together with Japan, these two Asian countries stand out as having relatively high male-contraceptive use statistics. Nonetheless, around the world, when couples want to prevent pregnancies, it is ordinarily the responsibility of the woman.

I once proposed a "couple" method that would allow the man and woman to alternate time intervals of taking an oral contraceptive. I thought that in addition to contraception, it would be a good sharing experience for husband and wife. The male pill I had in mind (gossypol) required a few months of use before sperm production stopped, so it would fit in nicely if the wife used the conventional pill during that interval.

We undertook some preliminary attitudinal surveys and found only a lukewarm response on the part of women in different cultures. Not infrequently, the American woman's response was along the line of, "Are you kidding? I can't even trust him to take out the garbage!"

In India, initially the idea received a positive response until we got to the question, "Would you agree to your husband taking a pill if it had the same health risks as the pill you would take?" That's where we lost them. "Health risk to my husband? No, no, certainly not!" Any risk to the husband was considered unacceptable to women in traditionally male-dominated Indian culture.

Health risks aside, today's contraceptives are not perfect. Even when couples have access to modern methods, contraceptive failure is not uncommon. Millions of women throughout the world, finding that their contraceptive method has failed to prevent an unwanted pregnancy, turn to abortion. When this is done under unsafe conditions, the woman's health is placed at risk. Tubal ligation is usually assumed to be the gold standard for effectiveness in preventing pregnancy, but it does not always succeed. During the first year after the surgery, about 4 women per 1000 will learn by having a pregnancy that the operation was not successful.

Among reversible methods, failure rates for one year of typical use are lowest with copper-carrying or progestin-releasing IUDs, contraceptive implants, or injectable progestins. This group of long-acting methods has a failure rate of less than 0.5% per year of use. The conventional pill, the mini-pill, and inert plastic IUDs are associated with a pregnancy rate of 3–5%. Failure rates with use of the condom, vaginal sponges or spermicides, cervical cap, diaphragm, rhythm, and withdrawal range from 12 to 21%.

It is a simple matter to calculate the number of pregnancies that result from contraceptive failure by multiplying the number of users of each method by its annual failure rate. It adds up to about 1.5 million. This calculation matches closely the survey data compiled by the National Center for Health Statistics.

Since roughly half of these pregnancies are voluntarily terminated, I can claim with confidence that there is no surer way to reduce the number of abortions in the United States and throughout the world than by improving the effectiveness of contraception. The World Health Organization recently completed a study concluding that if Chinese women had access to a highly effective emergency contraceptive (morning-after pill), abortions would be reduced by 40%.

If for no other reason, the less-than-satisfactory performance of currently available methods is a good reason for improved and more effective methods. I have never understood why there is not a natural alliance between those who preach for fewer abortions on Sunday and those who work every day of the year in the scientific search for contraceptive methods that are more effective. Opposition to both abortion and contraception has nothing to do with protecting the well-being of women and their families.

The choice of contraceptive methods available to American women is meager compared to the choice women have in European countries. The most recent U.S. Census Bureau's report on the subject reveals that the pill and the condom are the only nonsurgical contraceptives used to any significant extent. Methods popular in other countries like an array of IUDs, Depoprovera, and Norplant, as well as the diaphragm, rhythm, withdrawal, and vaginal spermicides all have a less than 2% rate of use, and some of them are barely mentioned at all in the surveys done to accumulate this information.

The Cairo Conference Plan of Action did not overlook this need. Recognizing the limited contraceptive options, the report called for governments and industry to significantly increase their support to bring new effective methods to market and to ensure the safety and quality of methods of regulating fertility. This call to action faces difficult barriers. Its chance of success is challenged by an underlying philosophy of how technology advances. Remember Dr. Doolittle's "push-me-pull-you"? This was the friendly beast that seemed to be going in two directions as the same time. Who was in charge? We have a similar dilemma in science. For new products, is the best strategy to define what is needed, and then try to pull scientific research along in that direction, or do advances in knowledge push product development toward what is scientifically feasible?

The toy industry is an example of product development by the "pull-you" method. Market research early in the year tells companies what will sell during the oncoming Christmas season. The product designers are then put to work cranking out what the public seems to want. The pharmaceutical industry, on the other hand, usually depends on the "push-me" approach. A new scientific breakthrough somewhere pushes the product development people into looking for a way to utilize the new knowledge for human application. A university scientist reports that the nonsteroidal anti-inflammatory drugs are based on the inhibition of two separate enzymes. If one of them is selectively inhibited, the anti-inflammatory action is maintained while lowering the risk of gastrointestinal bleeding associated with earlier products. Based on this solid science, the pharmaceutical industry is willing to undertake the investment of hundreds of millions of dollars to bring a new class of anti-inflammatory drugs to the market. This is why arthritis suffers now have the new blockbuster drugs, Celebrex and Vioxx.

Pharmaceutical companies do not make so large an investment carelessly. Seeking examples in medicine of success stories based on the toy company approach does not come up with a very long list. The polio vaccine did not emerge because Jonas Salk started out by saying, I am going to develop a polio vaccine. It happened because the science of vaccines reached a point of maturity and basic science finally had breakthroughs on the cause of the disease and how it is transmitted. Propelled forward by this information, Salk could make his final, valuable contribution to vaccine development. Chalk this up as a success for the push-me approach, even though some of the competition and jealousies of academic research probably delayed the vaccine for many summers. Disagreements among prestigious scientists prevented the funding of vaccine development until long after the facts had been assembled to move forward. Academia is not above human frailties. My friend Gerald Weissmann likes to quote the wry remark of Jack Whitehead, whose fortunes endowed the Whitehead Cancer Research Center at MIT. According to Whitehead, "in industry, it's dog eat dog; in academia, it is the opposite."

I hope we can avoid these problems as funding agencies attempt the heralded pull-you efforts to develop an AIDS vaccine. So far, there have been lots of hope and announcements but no vaccine. It would, indeed, be the world's greatest Christmas present, but it will happen only when the basic science of the virus and how to attack it within infected cells are better understood.

Oral contraceptives, IUDs, implants, and other delivery systems for hormonal steroids may seem like they were developed on demand to meet an identified need, but they were, in fact, pushed along by advances in organic chemistry, reproductive endocrinology, and related sciences. When Gregory Pincus was bluntly asked by Katherine McCormick and Margaret Sanger if he could develop the "perfect contraceptive," he hesitated before saying yes. I'm sure that under his breath he was adding "if the chemists make some breakthroughs, if Dr. Chang's laboratory can develop the right assay systems, if Dr. Rock's team confirms the laboratory results," and several other ifs as well. Science drives product development. Attempting to do catch-up science in order to develop a product is risky business.

There are many products that seem to replicate others already on the market, and their development absorbs a large part of the contraceptive research budget in industry. These "me-too" products are justified by their in-house advocates because of one or another advantage that can be pointed out to consumers in order to win their business. Over the years, for example, more than 50 oral contraceptive products followed the first one onto the market. In the process, doses were continuously lowered or new progestins were used. Consequently, the present forms of oral contraception have less than 1/20 the dose of the original product that reached the market, and the estrogen content is a small fraction of the original amount, without lowering effectiveness. These changes are marketed as safety or performance improvements.

The related field of assisted reproduction to treat infertility is referred to as the other side of the fertility control coin. It is a breathtaking story of public needs and scientific discoveries going in the same direction. Before 1960, assisted reproduction consisted of advising infertile couples to relax, attempts at artificial insemination with either husband or donor sperm, or rebound therapy. The first successful freezing and thawing of human sperm, by the addition of glycerol to prevent cell breakage, was heralded as a brave new world technological advance and led to the establishment of sperm banks backed by a few entrepreneurial investors.

The first case of a successful pregnancy outcome using thawed sperm was done at the University Hospital in Iowa City, with a $25 sperm sample provided by a medical student and standard laboratory supplies, supervised by Dr. Jerome Sherman, who was one of my classmates at Erasmus Hall High School in Brooklyn. Now, in the United States, the sale of assisted reproduction products alone is a $2.5-billion industry. Adding fees for service increases the total to almost $5 billion. The origins of this new, major industry were in bench science, such as Sherman's work on how to get sperm through the freezing step without having ice crystals rupture the sperm membrane. Dr. Luigi Mastroianni began studying in vitro fertilization requirements using the gametes of rhesus monkeys in the early 1960s. Isotope assays replaced tedious bioassays so that physicians could determine the hormone status of their patients, and receptor biology emerged and served as the basis for comparing potency and specificity of synthetic sex steroids.

In my New York laboratory we studied experimental drugs provided by the William S. Merrell Company of Cincinnati (now absorbed by pharmaceutical giant Aventis) that were modeled after the synthetic hormone stilbestrol (DES). We learned that the derivatives could prevent pregnancy in laboratory animals by accelerating the rate of passage of eggs in the fallopian tube. The late Dr. Robert Greenblatt of Augusta, renowned for his work in treating infertility, followed up on our laboratory studies, believing they might have the same action in humans and found that the two compounds, MER-25 and MRL-41, could induce ovulation in his patients.

One of these DES derivatives became Clomid, one of the successful fertility drugs still commonly in use. Compounds varying somewhat in structure from Clomid were synthesized and proved to be useful for the treatment of breast cancer and osteoporosis.

The other major fertility drug, Pergonal, came from research by the Italian company Serono Laboratories, in the process of seeking an immunological pregnancy test to replace the rabbit test. Led by biologist Pierro Donini, this work began the transition of Serona from a small local company concentrating on diagnostics, to a major multinational corporation and a leader in the pharmaceutical industry.

With specialized disposable equipment, expensive culture media, incubators, micromanipulators, and sophisticated microscopes, pretty soon you've got a multi-billion dollar industry. As a result, tens of thousands of couples have been able to overcome infertility problems and become parents.

As assisted reproduction flourished, advances in the field of contraception and voluntary fertility control have kept pace. New methods have been added, and older technologies, almost without exception, have been modified or improved. In the 1960s the debate concerning surgical tubal ligation was whether it was better to be done between pregnancies or immediately after delivery, when the fallopian tube is easily accessible. In either case it would require general anesthesia and abdominal surgery. Now, for the most part, it is an outpatient procedure using a laporascope. There is even a new device being studied that will be a non-incisional permanent tubal occlusion done through a hysteroscope. The sterilization operation for men has also been simplified. In China, where millions of vasectomies have been performed, it is referred to as the nonscalpel vasectomy.

Risky mercury-containing compounds, formerly used in vaginal spermicides, have been replaced by biological detergents, available in various delivery systems including creams, gels, films, sponges, or foams. Condoms are now sold in a variety of colors and textures, and replacing latex with a self-lubricating plastic has increased impermeability. There is now available in some countries a female condom, which is intended to improve the protection for women against sexually transmitted diseases, including HIV. Even the rhythm method is no longer simply the calendar or temperature method (or fertility beads), but can be used in conjunction with a sophisticated instrument that measures daily rates of change in a woman's endocrine profile.

But the major contraceptive market has been orally active hormones that can safely inhibit ovulation. Oral contraceptives accounted for nearly $3 billion of the world total contraceptive market of $4.0 billion in 2000. At the peak, 36 companies worldwide were marketing more than 50 brand names of the pill and 12 mini-pills. The United States accounts for more than half of the worldwide revenues in contraceptives. The next largest is Europe with about $750 million. Japan's market is growing now that the pill has been approved for use as a contraceptive. Estimates are that its total dollar sales will soon equal or exceed Europe's. Condom sales account for about $250 million, and spermicides, diaphragms, IUDs, injectables, and Norplant add another quarter billion dollars of sales globally.

The developing world's contraceptive use has been growing steadily and now stands at about 600 million users of either traditional or modern methods. The United Nations estimates that by 2007, when the world will have nearly 1 billion more people than the current 6 billion plus, there will be more than 750 million couples in developing countries using contraceptives. The UN projects that from 1997 to 2007, the developing world will use over 12 billion cycles of the pill, 70 billion condoms, 900 million contraceptive injections, 436 million IUDs, and nearly 20 million subdermal contraceptive implants, and that the grand total for this shopping cart of contraceptives will be $9 billion.

Although contraceptive use has increased steadily over the past decades and the global market is bound to grow further, there are several indications that consumers would welcome still better products. More than 50% of the 6 million pregnancies in the United States each year are unintended at the time of conception. Half of these occur when no contraception is being used. The other half of these unintended pregnancies occur while a couple is attempting to use a contraceptive method. A similar situation prevails globally. In Japan, for example, where condom use is very high, fully 64% of all pregnancies annually are classified as "accidents." Latin America is another striking example of the inadequacy of present contraception's performance or accessibility. Women describe only 38% of the region's 16 million annual pregnancies as wanted at the time of conception. About half of unplanned pregnancies are carried to term, and the other half terminate with abortion.

In the United States, each year about 1.5 million of the 32 million women who use contraceptives learn by a positive pregnancy test that the method they chose didn't work for them. Half of these disappointed women elect to have an abortion. Globally, the number of unplanned pregnancies following contraceptive failure cannot be calculated with equal precision, but based on the best available data, the number is between 40 and 80 million.

Another problem is that discontinuation of use rates are high for most methods. Contraceptive users tend to switch from method to method in an effort to find one that is best for them. In the United States, one out of four users of oral contraceptives discontinue its use before the end of one year. The rate is even higher for teenage users. About 50% of women using the vaginal sponge and other barrier methods do not complete the first year of use, and 60% of condom users switch within a year to another method. For women who start the injectable contraceptive, DepoProvera, 50% discontinue before the end of the first year. Long-acting methods, such as the IUD and Norplant, have one-year continuation of use rates in the 90% range. Facilitating this high rate of continuation is the fact that to discontinue requires going to a clinic or a doctor's office.

Surgical sterilization is the most widely used method of fertility regulation around the world. In the United States, tubal ligation and vasectomy combined account for 36% of contraceptive use, followed by oral contraceptives at 15%, condom use at 11%, and other methods far behind. Many who select the surgical methods do so because they believe they have completed their family size and opt for the near-certainty of the operation. But others elect to have the usually irreversible operation because of their disappointment with the alternative choices that are available to them. This is happening at younger and younger age. Consequently, there is a growing demand for reversal operations as life situations change and the restoration of fertility becomes important. Worldwide figures and trends are similar; women are seeking tubal ligation at earlier ages. Dissatisfaction with the features of reversible methods now available and their side effects contributes to the decision to seek the surgical alternative.

There are new priorities expected of contraceptive methods. Younger couples entering their reproductive years want protection against sexually transmitted diseases, including HIV, greater control of their contraception rather than depending on clinic services, and the opportunity for men to share in the responsibility of contraception.

In spite of the expanding global market and evidence of consumer interest in new products, discovery and development in the field of fertility control does not have high priority in the established pharmaceutical industry. Ordinarily, when the science is ripe and there is a demand for a product, companies support research and development and enter the market. But most major companies are not interested in contraceptive product development. There is some product development activity in the field but rarely by major companies that have the resources required for a full-scale effort. According to an FDA official who scanned the nonconfidential information available on the subject, in 1996, there were 50 investigational new drug applications (INDs) active in the United States. They included work on new oral contraceptives, implants, injectables, delivery systems for hormones (transdermal and vaginal rings), a new IUD, and vaginal microbicides. Most of these were variations on existing methods or initiatives of publicly supported research programs that had not identified commercial partners for full product development and marketing activities.

Five years later, most of these INDs had been abandoned, and patents on ideas for contraceptive products were not being pursued. Paradoxically, as I have described in the preceding chapter, the three-year period from 2000 to 2002 produced a record number of contraceptive product launches in the United States. A few are industry-initiated, but these are chiefly products that were developed by publicly supported programs and not by pharmaceutical company product development efforts. As the leads these programs are working on run out, the negative effect of large company not participating in the field will take effect.

The appeal of the Cairo conference notwithstanding, it is likely that large pharmaceutical companies will remain on the sidelines. Corporations do not view themselves as instruments of social change. They are in business to make money. If, concurrently, they can do good, that's fine, but doing good is not what drives corporate decision-making. In most companies, an internal advocate for a product with potential return equal to or even less than that of a new contraceptive will prevail in the competition for a share of the company's research budget. This decision is understandable because it allows the company to maintain a pipeline of new products while avoiding the "rage factor" from opponents of reproductive choice.

The "rage factor" is the aggregate of complaints, harassment, and threats that may be directed toward a company identified with a particular type of product. Boycott threats are no longer the extreme in this category. Death threats to individual officers or their families and terrorist bombing threats against an entire factory have also become a reality for companies considering products that radical opponents object to, specifically in the realm of reproductive choice. Sad to say, these anonymous terrorists are successful in their efforts to frighten companies and influence the research agenda.

No other cause elicits comparable rage response, even though there are issues that prompt opposition to particular products. For Wyeth-Ayerst, for example, the protests of animal groups about the use of bodily fluids from horses for the preparation of Premarin is a bearable burden, considering that Premarin has been the largest selling prescription drug for women's health in the United States and the envy of the entire industry.

In the United States companies have to consider the additional problem of concern about liability issues. All too often, the history of reproductive health products can be described as from laboratory bench to bedside and back to the bench—the judge's bench.

Consumer advocacy groups and the plaintiff's bar in the United States believe that the country's litigious atmosphere, with respect to contraceptive product liability, cannot be held responsible for the failure of pharmaceutical companies to give higher priority to contraceptive development. Their view is that it is not lawyers who drove contraceptives off the market, but drug companies who put defective products on the market. The example usually cited is the class action suit involving the Dalkon Shield. This was, indeed, a faulty product and deserved to be driven from the market. In fact, this is the only contraceptive drug or device no longer marketed because of a legal action requiring that it be withdrawn. As the lawyers might say, the Dalkon Shield case is *sui generis*.

In 1973, the Centers for Disease Control and Prevention in Atlanta began to receive reports of mid-trimester deaths associated with infection and the use of the Dalkon Shield, an IUD marketed by the A.H. Robins Company. In 1974 an analysis of the data confirmed the association. By then more than 3 million American women were using the Dalkon Shield. The product was withdrawn from the American market immediately after the initial reports of device-associated deaths, but the company continued to market the device abroad for almost a year. By 1984 juries in eight cases had imposed a total of more than $17 million in punitive damages, and there were 3500 pending cases, which also demanded punitive damages. In 1985 the A.H. Robins Company filed for bankruptcy in violation of an agreement it had with a key judge in the proceedings. Ever since, the case has been cited as an example of a contraceptive-marketing company hounded into bankruptcy by overzealous lawyers. To the contrary, the fate of the Dalkon Shield and its sponsoring company was well deserved and stands as a good example of the consumer protection offered by adverse reaction reporting to the Centers for Disease Control, surveillance by FDA of prescription products, and the U.S. legal system.

The problem is that in an episode like this, there is a ripple effect. The impact of litigation against contraceptive products can be more extensive than the fate of the individual product involved. After the Dalkon Shield judgment, the successful lawyers transferred their attention to the copper-T IUDs, for which there was no scientific evidence of harm to users, faulty design, or any other basis for product liability claims. The cost of defense and the burden on the legal departments of the affected companies (G.D. Searle and Ortho) led them to withdraw their products. The real losers were American women who, for many years afterwards, had only limited access to devices effectively and safely used elsewhere in the world.

The Norplant legal woes also had a broad negative impact, although all the plaintiffs' claims against Norplant were refuted by substantial scientific evidence. The negative publicity generated by the litigation drastically damaged sales in the United States and chilled the atmosphere for introducing implant contraceptives elsewhere. Wyeth International never introduced Norplant into the French market, despite receiving regulatory agency approval for its use in France. Another distributor withdrew Norplant from the United Kingdom in spite of its initial financial success, and the parent company, Wyeth-Ayerst, is undecided on the introduction of an FDA-approved, second-generation implant system, Jadelle, in the United States. Théramex, a European company, was well on the way to having the first single-implant product on the market when they withdrew from a joint development partnership. When the Monaco-based company was bought out by the German Merck company, the contraceptive implant product was buried.

The FDA approved the Norplant contraceptive implant system in 1991, after it had been distributed commercially in Europe and elsewhere for a decade. By 1997 more than 7 million Norplant contraceptives had been distributed worldwide, and more than 1 million women in the United States had adopted this long-acting method of contraception. After the U.S. launch, Norplant soon began to encounter litigation problems. More than 200 lawsuits, at least 50 of which were class actions, were filed against Wyeth-Ayerst, the distributing company. Ultimately, not a single case was successful, including a case before a district court in Louisiana, a venue presumably chosen by the plaintiff's attorney because of the reputation of the elected judge to favor certifying class action suits. In the U.S. tort law system, it is of no consequence that there has never been an adverse reaction to Norplant use reported to the Centers for Disease Control and Prevention from the entire state of Louisiana. The plaintiff's lawyer can search for a favorable courthouse to plead his case.

It is not an overstatement to say that the liability issue is the biggest roadblock to contraceptive product development in the United States. Insurance costs, unwillingness to cannibalize existing markets, and company image also play a role. Nevertheless, it is noteworthy that in the 1990s there were 20,000 product liability suits (for all products, not just contraceptives) annually in the United States and only 200 in the United Kingdom. Obviously, product liability litigation is a thriving industry in the United States at a level unmatched in the United Kingdom and other European countries. General features of the American legal system are far more influential than actual differences in laws in explaining the enormous difference between the number and costs of product liability cases in the United States as compared to Europe. The real differences lie in rules governing such matters as trial by jury, pretrial discovery, the system of paying lawyers (contingent fee arrangements are not allowed in Europe), use of expert witnesses, selection of jurisdiction, and the procedures by which judges are seated.

The battle of experts, a familiar part of product liability lawsuits in the United States, contrasts with the presentation of scientific evidence in Europe. Product liability cases frequently turn on the weight given to the testimony of expert witnesses. Partisan testimony that can impress jury members might carry less weight with a professional judge, who is the trier-of-fact in civil law cases in other countries. "Junk science," a commonplace feature of American tort trials, has not yet crossed the Atlantic. Under the European civil law system, a judge may designate the experts who will testify. Even if a party is given the privilege to select a witness to testify about scientific issues, it would be improper for the lawyer to consult with the expert before the trial. For an American lawyer not to prepare a friendly expert witness would be unthinkable; in the civil law of countries in Europe such preparation would be considered unethical.

The liability history of contraceptive drugs and devices in the United States is extensive. The pill, the IUD, injectables, implants, and even spermicides have come under fire from the plaintiff's bar. Some see this history as proof that contraceptive products tend to be singled out for legal attack, but perhaps this is an exaggeration. There are other examples of legal battles involving women's health products such as bendectin (used for morning sickness), stilbestrol, thalidomide, and silicone breast implants. In some of these examples the claims of injury were clearly justified, but in others the weight of scientific evidence did not support claims. It is difficult to escape the conclusion that interventions involving the reproductive system are held to different standards or elicit different emotional responses than other pharmaceutical products or devices.

The lesson is inescapable that research on human reproduction, along the entire pathway from bench science to product introduction, must adhere to the highest level of ethical and scientific standards. There are no short cuts in science, in general. Reproduction research, like Caesar's wife, must be beyond reproach.

The benefits of contraception are becoming more universally available, but there remains a substantial unmet need throughout the world. Where there is unmet demand, women's right to reproductive freedom continues to be denied. It is a freedom so much taken for granted by those who have it that sometimes we tend to forget how vital it can be in the lives of others who do not have it. Without effective and safe contraceptive methods, women cannot have the opportunity to fulfill their roles as mothers in balance with personal goals that are open to men. They cannot gain control over their lives and over the hopes and aspirations for their children. Barriers to further advances in contraception should fall, not for the sake of enriching pharmaceutical companies, but to provide women with even better methods than the inadequate contraceptive technology that we have today. I have testified on this subject before congressional committees with members who just don't get it and have given public lectures under harassment by ignorant fanatics. On one occasion, the Baltimore police department had to physically remove two threatening individuals who attempted to shut down our panel discussion on technology at an International Student's Pugwash conference. The terrorists, bullies, and ideologues cannot be allowed to take over public discourse or set the research agenda for contraceptive advances.

8

Feeding the World's People

Controversy tends to keep topics and personalities in the public eye. Who would remember Thomas Robert Malthus, an eighteenth-century English cleric destined for obscurity, had he not published one of the most controversial articles of all time? In 1798 he predicted that population growth would soon outstrip food supply because, he wrote: "The power of population is infinitely greater than the power of the earth to produce subsistence for man." Human populations, he claimed, tend to increase exponentially, while food supplies increase linearly. A Cambridge-trained economist, his ideas were somewhat more complex, but the basic Malthusian idea, exponential versus linear, has been taught to high school and college students for more than 200 years.

The nineteenth and twentieth centuries appeared to prove that Malthus was wrong. Population size has, indeed, increased almost exponentially from the time of his world of less than 1 billion to today's 6 billion people, but food supply has kept up. If there is a Malthusian race between food and population, food has been winning. Food has maintained its lead in spite of the fact that there was record population growth in the last half of the twentieth century. Disagreement on the

144

subject seems never to end. Nowadays, to be labeled "neo-Malthusian" carries a certain stigma of fanaticism concerning population growth. The next sentence usually adds the moniker "prophet of gloom."

Wagering against the gloomy predictions of imminent famine could have been a profitable hobby. Respected biologist Paul Ehrlich wrote in 1976 that feeding a population of 6 billion would be impossible. The agricultural economist brother team, William and Paul Paddock, captured headlines with their book, *Famine, 1975!* So far, these predictions of disaster have all turned out to be wrong. Hidden behind the international system of supplementary food supplies to avert large-scale famine, however, there are many people in the world who do not get adequate food and are chronically malnourished—not for Malthusian reasons but because of the short comings of the world's food distribution systems.

The status of the food–population race depends on the stakes. If you were betting against the predictions of mass starvation, you would have won. If you bet that there would not be hunger and malnutrition, you would have lost. Food supplies and distribution may have prevented the mass famines that have been predicted, but they have not been sufficient to keep people adequately fed. Some years were cliffhangers. India in the 1960s, after consecutive years of draught, had to be fed with millions of tons of grains rushed from United States granaries. Quite literally India's people were being fed from ship to mouth. More recently, we have seen the heartbreaking pictures of starving children in Somalia scrambling for a few grains of rice while warring militia forces were stealing the relief supplies that had been shipped there.

A United Nations conference in 1996 concluded that nearly 800 million people, greater than 13% of the world's population, were chronically hungry and malnourished. The situation is not improving. At the end of the twentieth century, the estimate of numbers of malnourished people had increased, and officials of the UN's Food and Agriculture Organization had to back off the pledge to eliminate malnutrition and adopt a less ambitious goal to reduce it by half in 10 years.

Disproportionately, the chronically malnourished are in Africa. The United Nations estimates that in sub-Saharan Africa 33% of the population is undernourished. For many, particularly children, malnutrition leads to death because of increased vulnerability to disease. In the world's poorest countries, 400 million malnourished women of childbearing age suffer from iron-deficiency anemia that reduces the blood's oxygen-carrying capacity. Anemic women are more likely to die during pregnancy or to produce underweight babies. These babies have difficulty catching up in mental or physical development, particularly if they are born into circumstances of chronic malnutrition. The number of underweight babies in the world's less-developed countries is increasing with each passing decade.

Adequate food for the hungry is more complicated than production alone. Insufficient food to avoid hunger and starvation is a combination of the result of poverty, political instability and military conflict, distribution inequity, competition of highly subsidized farm products, land ownership policies, and natural disasters, as well as production shortfalls.

Over the course of history, as demand for food has increased, people have staved off starvation by finding ingenious ways to create new land to place under cultivation. Moving the frontiers of civilization, terracing hillsides, and draining swamp land have all accomplished this purpose. Even pushing back the sea has worked to reclaim more land for farming.

By the mid-twentieth century, the limit for large-scale cropland expansion had just about been reached. There were no new continents to discover or vast virgin territories to explore. The last major increase occurred when the plains of Kazakhstan, on the eastern edge of the then-Soviet Union, were converted to farmland in the 1950s. This brought and for wheat farming under cultivation equivalent to the capacity of Canada and Australia combined.

There was another surge in cultivated acreage in the 1970s and 1980s when farmers pushed the limits of their holdings to take advantage of the rising price of wheat, but by then they were plowing marginal land that could not be cultivated year after year. Even the new croplands of Kazakhstan have this serious limitation. Soil management experts believe that the initial bonanza of 25 million hectares will eventual shrink to about half that area of usable cropland.

With scant opportunity for increases in farmland to feed the world's growing population, Malthus might have had the last word, after all, had food production not found some other means to keep pace. Science came to the rescue with amazing advances in crop yields per acre, achieved through classical plant-breeding techniques and the intensive use of fertilizers, pesticides, and irrigation.

This achievement was the aptly named the "Green Revolution," fostered by a cooperative effort of industrialized and developing nations, richly funded by a number of governmental and foundation sources. Research centers were set up where there was a need for greater food output: wheat and maize research in Mexico, rice research in the Philippines, forestry and livestock research in Kenya. During the years of the Cold War, the world lived consciously with the day-to-day efforts to maintain peace, sometimes coming close to breaking down. A quiet struggle was going on simultaneously to avert the disaster of global instability that could be caused by massive food shortages. The success was phenomenal. New varieties of rice, wheat, and corn that increased per-acre yields dramatically were developed in record time. These are the crops that sustain the earth's people.

As the world's population grew from 2.5 billion in 1950 to 6 billion, food supplies kept up. The new miracle seeds raised production of grains and cereals, crops that provide at least 80% of food worldwide and that feed most of the world's people. From 1950 to 1990 world grain yield per acre increased steadily. In the Gangetic plain of northern India, the introduction of new varieties of wheat increased yields up to sevenfold. Rice yields in Asia increased from 1 ton per hectare to 8 tons per hectare. Corn production was increased to four times what farmers were accustomed to. Science could take credit for these substantial gains, but they were possible only because of the willingness of indigenous farmers everywhere to break with tradition and adopt new ways to grow their crops.

In 1997, the United Nation's Food and Agriculture Organization was able to report that, in spite of the huge increase in population of the developing world, overall food per capita had increased by 20% since the 1960s. Widespread famine was averted. Nevertheless, there are still 800 million hungry people in these regions, many of them seriously malnourished preschool children. Moreover, some developing countries are still dependent on imported food, making them precariously vulnerable to conditions outside their control. A serious drought or political turmoil can place entire populations in jeopardy. Somalia in the 1990s would have been a scene of even worse conditions of starvation without the foreign food shipments mentioned earlier. By 2001, the four years of drought in Afghanistan had driven millions from their homes and created a nation of refugees, dependent on the United Nations and other outside agencies to stave off mass starvation.

The 1977 award of the Nobel Prize for the Promotion of Peace went to agricultural scientist Norman Borlaug for his role in the Green Revolution. This recognition of a man of science acknowledged that technological advances had averted a disaster as the world headed toward a chaotic food crisis. When I congratulated Borlaug, he was characteristically blunt in reminding me that the Green Revolution simply bought some time, but that it should not engender complacency about the ability to feed future generations of a rapidly growing population.

While Borlaug was leading wheat and maize research in Mexico, Robert Chandler was the founding director of the International Rice Research Institute (IRRI) in the Philippines. It was at IRRI that high-yield rice varieties were developed, destined to feed most of Asia through the last half of the twentieth century. Like Borlaug, Chandler has always glanced over his shoulder, fearful of the world's inability to feed growing numbers of people. In 1990, when Bangladesh had a population of about 60 million, Chandler wrote in reaction to the World Bank's population growth projection for that country: "More than half of the rural population is landless and is severely underemployed. Over 70% of the farms are less than one hectare in size. I cannot conceive of Bangladesh supporting the number of people predicted." By 2000 the population of Bangladesh had grown to 129 million, heading on the predicted track toward 200 million shortly after 2025. Food production is barely keeping pace with population growth, and the number of children underweight remains well above 50%.

China's agricultural research program independently succeeded in breeding high-yield varieties of rice during the 1950s. Turned inward during that period of the ancient country's history, its science was essentially closed off from the rest of the world's scientific community. Years later, when Western agriculture experts learned that Chinese plant breeders had developed a variety of dwarf rice identical to the high-yield seeds developed at IRRI they were eager to compare experiences.

Sterling Wortman, a Rockefeller Foundation agricultural scientist, told me about a visit to China shortly after relations improved and scientists began to exchange information. The visitors asked what had happened in China in certain years when much of the IRRI variety rice crop had been lost in spite of abundant application of pesticides. There was scientific interest in learning if the infestation of the brown planthopper, which had caused most of the devastation, had spread to the territories where China had planted with their new variety. The Western agronomists were surprised to learn that China had escaped these losses. The reason was simple. According to a 2000-year-old proverb, Chinese rice farmers have known that "the spider is the friend of the paddy." So, when they saw that the level of fertilizer and pesticides required for the new rice variety killed off the spiders, they intuitively cut back on the amounts, permitting the spiders to survive even though the resultant crop yields were not optimal. Saving the spiders had prevented the sucking brown planthopper from taking over the paddies because the spider is its natural enemy. This was a case of modern technology learning something from centuries-old traditional agriculture. Robert Herdt, the agricultural economist who now holds the Rockefeller Foundation's vice presidency occupied by Wortman 25 years ago, told me recently that China's performance on this issue has changed dramatically in a quarter century. Now Chinese farmers are the world's most extravagant users of pesticides and fertilizers, raising their rice in virtually sterile paddies. Although some rice diseases remain resistant, China has one of the world's highest rice yields. Chemical additives have replaced the spider as the Chinese rice farmer's best friend. Nevertheless, in China and elsewhere in Asia, biotechnology researchers hopefully screen rice varieties for natural resistance to the planthopper. Perhaps they need to be reminded that the spider is the friend of the paddy.

The food–population race is not over. One does not have to be a neo-Malthusian to acknowledge that 30 years from now there will be an extra 2.5 billion people in poor countries in need of food. The momentum of population growth cannot be stopped in this period, so increasing food production and assuring more equity in its distribution must be the plan of action. The world's farmers have to be able to produce more, and poor people need to have the means to buy food. If this is not achieved, the gains of the past will be lost, and the number of malnourished and hungry will grow. Growth in the world's demand for grain is driven both by the increase in population numbers and by the rise in affluence that is enabling so many of the world's low-income consumers to move up the food chain, eating more grain-intensive meat and dairy products.

Estimates by agricultural experts indicate that to continue feeding the world's growing population at its present nutritional level, food production will have to double by 2030. This demand comes at a time when yields per acre are not maintaining their robust growth of the recent past, and there is no realistic outlook for expansion of farm acreage. In fact, there has been serious loss of croplands, and this trend will continue. Moreover, shortage of fresh water prohibits major expansion of agricultural irrigation, which is needed for high yields.

The peak of world grain-producing area was reached in 1981. It has since fallen almost 10% and will decline further as marginal lands under cultivation become unusable. The bitter harvest of intense farming is land degradation, as topsoil is lost through water or wind erosion. Nutrients that took scores of years to accumulate in rich soil can be lost in one plowing and planting season. This was what prompted the soil scientist Daniel Hillel to write that "the plowshare has been far more destructive than the sword." With plowing and cultivation, topsoil is not lost if it simply moves from one farming area to another, but frequently this irreplaceable resource ends up as silt in river or lake beds. Agricultural land acreage lost and population increase have caused the ratio of world grain-land per person to fall almost 50% in the last 20 years, continuing a decline that has been evident since 1950.

The relationship between food and population is more complex than supply and demand. People have to be able to purchase food. Except to stave off famine in emergencies, no one gives it away. Food gifting cannot go on indefinitely. It discourages local producers or even drives them out of business if they have to compete with highly subsidized or free distribution of the products they are trying to sell to make a living. Governments have to establish farm policies that encourage growers to plant high-yielding varieties of grains and other sustenance crops. On the macro scale, governments cannot afford to allow a country's food supply to become dependent on external sources. Around the world, food security is politically essential. Uncertainty about a secure food supply can be a serious threat to political stability. And the corollary is also true: Political chaos is a threat to food security.

There is also the microeconomics of food and population. I remember a farmer in Puebla, Mexico, who provided a graphic example. During a visit by Rockefeller Foundation officials, he thanked the foundation for its help in introducing high-yield wheat that had been developed at Borlaug's nearby research center. He explained that without the increased yields, he and his family could not have afforded to stay and work the land. Father Ted Hesburgh, the multilingual president of Notre Dame University and the foundation's chairman at the time, asked the farmer how many children he had. The proud answer was that he had four sons and three daughters. He volunteered, however, that he had a dilemma. The family could not divide the land among his sons (like the Bombay doctor I mentioned earlier he didn't mention his daughters) and remain efficient producers. Only the oldest son farmed with him. To avoid breaking up the land into smaller farms, the other three had moved into Mexico City to seek urban jobs. As population size increases, this farmer's dilemma is one of the causes of the massive shift of population from rural to urban life throughout the world.

The world is on the threshold of the largest food demand in human history. Inevitably, food production will have to double. However, over the past 2 decades, more than 300,000 square miles of land that was previously in farming have been lost to urban expansion and other uses. The United States alone has paved over more cropland than the area of New Jersey. In the gold rush to build new shopping malls, highways, golf courses, and parking lots, fertile land seemed expendable because yield increases per acre became the principal means for increasing food production. In fact, U.S. food production increased more rapidly than the demand for it. When in the mid-1960s I moved my family into our tiny community in Westchester County, just half an hour from the New York City limits, one of the bucolic appeals was an egg farm within walking distance and a small vegetable farm just a few minutes away. Now, the egg farm is gone to make way for an interstate highway and the vegetable farm has sold out to a golf driving range. This a trivial but personal example is what the entire world is experiencing.

As new crop varieties, pesticides, and the increased use of fertilizer and irrigation made each acre more productive, rising yields became a strikingly effective substitute for land expansion. Production not only kept up with the rising demands of billions more people, it even outpaced population growth. Food surpluses grew in some countries, increasing the list of food exporters. The price of food staples has fallen dramatically. During the last half of the twentieth-century, the prices, in constant dollars, of wheat and corn dropped more than 50%. Whether this can continue is the subject of debate. Will the negative effects of intensified farming drain the soil resources before agroscientists discover how to replenish soil nutrients?

Farmers in the United States and China have achieved most of the great increases in grain yield per acre. Together these countries produce more than 40% of the world's grain, and they have raised their average from 1 to nearly 5 tons of grain per hectare. Fueling these impressive gains was the lavish use of fertilizers and abundant irrigation of croplands. This may have been a winning combination in the recent past, but it is also a recipe for danger ahead; each component cannot be counted on to meet future needs.

Each harvested acre will need to double its yield just to provide current nutritional levels for the projected population in 2030. This will never happen without new scientific breakthroughs. Agricultural experts do not believe that grain yields can be significantly increased by the conventional breeding techniques responsible for the Green Revolution. This is the first warning signal. The needed breakthroughs will have to be based on new science and the promising results achieved in biotechnology and genetic modification of foodstuffs. Higher yields will be possible if strains can be developed with genetic characteristics such as resistance to drought, frost, or disease. This is the second warning signal because genetic modification of foodstuffs faces stiff opposition unless these foods are proved to be absolute safe to both people and the environment.

In the research done so far, rice has been the pivotal plant. All grains share many identical chromosome segments with rice. This means that genetic research discoveries on rice are likely to be applicable to the entire group. In studies done at experimental agricultural stations, genes from wild species of rice have been identified that, when introduced to elite varieties, increase yields by some 20%. Researchers expected wild rice genes to be useful for imparting disease resistance. Increasing yields was a bonus in this genetic modification.

Chinese scientists have already developed new high-yield rice that breeds true for combined traits to resist disease and tolerate cold and drought. This new variety produces up to 24% higher yields. Because this type of research does not introduce foreign genes into rice plants, it can be interpreted as a way to fast-forward conventional plant breeding.

Food policy managers in countries at risk for food shortages are taking the initiative. In the Ivory Coast, scientists working in the West African Rice Development Association (WARDA), a sister institution to IRRI, the center in the Philippines I mentioned earlier, have crossbred Asian and African rice strains by using sophisticated tissue culture procedures. From this basic cross they have derived thousands of new varieties that local farmers can choose from to get the best growing properties for their paddies. The Ivory Coast will save billions in the cost of importing rice, and poor farmers will participate in assuring food security for the years ahead.

Plant biotechnology research is following different approaches. Some plants, such as corn, are called C-4 plants because they have the enzymes to produce four-carbon organic molecules as a first step in taking carbon dioxide out the atmosphere. This is an efficient way to produce organic matter from carbon dioxide fixation. Rice and wheat are C-3 plants because their first fixation product is a three-carbon organic molecule, which involves a more energy-intensive pathway to produce organic material. Consequently, the C-3 system produces about half as much grain protein per carbon dioxide fixed as C-4 plants. Scientists are trying to isolate and transfer the genes controlling the more efficient enzyme system. If successful, such genetic modification could result in almost doubling yields of present varieties of wheat and rice, provided the new gene construct proves to be harmless to consumers and to the environment.

Gene transfer is not the only tool in the hands of agricultural biotechnology scientists. Any method by which hereditary information can be transferred from one variety of plant to another is on the research agenda, and some of the potential results are amazing. Plant scientists can take the entire cytoplasm of one cell and chemically fuse it with another so that the hybrid cells formed may then regenerate into a whole plant incorporating the transferred hereditary information. This is the plant-world equivalent to cloning. Specific organelles within a plant cell such as chloroplasts or mitochondria can be moved to another cell, along with the specific hereditary information they possess. These techniques will have an enormous influence on plant breeding because a number of important traits, including herbicide tolerance, are controlled by cytoplasmic and organelle factors. This can be the pathway to the "Doubly Green Revolution" called for by Gordon Conway, the ecologist president of the Rockefeller Foundation. He foresees the great importance of new varieties of high-yield crops that conserve the use of water and do not stress the environment by high requirements for fertilizer, pesticides, or herbicidal chemicals.

The "golden rice" debate is an example of disagreements and misrepresentations that characterize the debate over genetic modification of foodstuffs. Vitamin A-deficiency disorders afflict billions of children and pregnant women in the world's poorest countries. Scientists have been able to introduce genes into rice plants that result in the production of beta-carotene, which gives the rice grain a golden hue. The human body converts beta-carotene into vitamin A. Therefore, golden rice could serve to supplement vitamin A-deficient diets in the same way that iodized salt is used to supplement iodine-deficient diets. The first golden rice varieties developed in the laboratory, if substituted for ordinary rice in the diet of poor people around the world, could contribute up to 20% of the daily requirements of vitamin A, and scientists are working on gene constructs that would increase the yield and avoid possible environmental hazards when the new varieties are released for planting. It will probably be 2005 before these new rice varieties would be available to farmers for field testing.

Media reports tend to exaggerate what the scientific community expects from golden rice and mislead the public with respect to the stage of its development. Critics of genetic modification also distort the facts in expressing their opposition. Taking the high ground, the environmental group Greenpeace, for example, says it prefers a complete balanced diet as a solution to vitamin A deficiency. Who doesn't? Golden rice is not expected to substitute for a balanced diet as the main source of vitamin A. Rather, it can provide a complement to fruits, vegetables, and animal products in the diet and can be particularly beneficial to those who can rarely, if ever, afford these essential foodstuffs. Opponents also express alarm that the new variety is just around the corner and that it will be introduced without adequate testing of environmental hazards and other dangers. A Greenpeace spokesperson said that the genetic engineering industry "is using the misery of mothers and children who suffer from [vitamin A deficiency] for its own commercial gain." This type of incendiary rhetoric is not helpful, nor are the violent attacks on test acreages that have driven test plantings into bomb-proof greenhouses.

I have discussed golden rice and genetic modification of foodstuffs with well-informed agro-ecologists and conclude that disagreements will be difficult to resolve. The basis of opposition goes far beyond genetic modification per se. For some, attitudes toward increasing food production through biotechnology are shaded by strongly held views concerning social injustice and poverty, globalization, free-market economy, land reform, private enterprise, and distrust of large agro-industries. Long-held positions on these issues will not soften easily, and as long as genetic food modification is the symbol and surrogate for this panoply of concerns, it will not be allowed either to move forward on its own merits or be held back because of its own deficiencies.

These disagreements are going to require greater willingness to understand and cooperate. Unlike the classical plant breeding of the first Green Revolution which was based on science in the public domain, the new advances will evolve in the changed atmosphere of patents, exclusivity, and science sponsored chiefly by agro-industry. This change in sponsorship raises suspicions among ecologists and environmentalists that, in the race for profits, companies may disregard hazards that could damage the earth's ecosystems, perhaps in irreversible ways, as genetically altered plants are released for agricultural use. There is concern, for example, that plants with an inserted gene to provide protection by producing an insect toxin might accelerate the rise of resistant pest insect populations and also kill nonpest insects such as the Monarch butterfly. And social activists are convinced that the poor peasant farmers around the globe will not benefit but be victimized by the new-world agriculture they see looming ahead. They will be competing with high technology mass producers using their labor-intensive, low-yield traditional farming methods.

Opponents to improving crop yield through advances in biotechnology need to offer feasible alternatives. Can future world food needs be met by means other than research and development of new varieties of high-yield, low-maintenance crops? Some believe that better management, not greater yield, is the solution. This is what Archer Daniels Midland used to say every night in its commercial supporting "News Hour with Jim Lehrer" on U.S. public television. "We can feed the world with the food we produce. What we need is better distribution of the food we now have." On the opposite end of the political spectrum, you hear the same message from land-reform activists who call for the break-up of large commercial farms and have organized landless families to move into millions of acres of land throughout Brazil and elsewhere. They would add the caveat that we can feed the world with present food if it is distributed fairly.

While I favor fairness, I am skeptical that relying on distribution reform is adequate assurance for tomorrow's food security. Some argue that farm subsidies in the West unfairly place local farmers in poor countries at an impossible competitive disadvantage, so that dropping farm subsidies in North America and Europe or providing equivalent support to farmers in poor countries would level the playing field. But the problem is far more complicated. Will the wheat farmers of the Punjab share their crop with Bihar's malnourished millions, rather than sell it in a lucrative export market destined for affluent countries? Who is going to compel farmers to grow the crops that the world needs, rather than the cash crops they want to grow on their own land? Will the newly redistributed land in Zimbabwe profitably producing cut flowers for the flower stalls of Europe be converted to grain production for local consumption? And who is going to prohibit feeding grain to animals because dairy and meat products waste grain calories?

Agriculture's need for abundant water carries the next uncertainty. Once considered an unlimited resource, water is becoming a scarce and valuable commodity. If the spider is a friend of the paddy, its *best* friend is water. The rice paddy is totally dependent on adequate supplies of fresh water. Rice, the world's most widely used grain, is also the most water dependent. On the average, producing a ton of harvested rice consumes a minimum of 1000 tons of water.

Some smart agronomist has calculated that just meeting the grain requirement of the projected world population in 2025 will need an additional 780 billion cubic meters of water. Adding the water requirements for the rest of a normal diet raises the total to more than 1000 billion cubic meters. This is the amount of fresh water needed just to feed at today's nutritional level the present 6 billion plus the 2.5 billion people who will be added in the first quarter of the new century. Forty percent of the world's total fresh water would need to be used to meet the grain requirement in 2025.

Today, countries fight over land. Some of these disputes are more about water than land, and these water conflicts are bound to intensify. At the Earth Summit in Johannesburg it was disclosed that about 1 billion people are without access to clean water. Nearly half the world's land area falls within international water basins shared by two or more countries. The threat of water wars between countries vying for dwindling water supplies will increase as the world's population grows and fresh water areas are wasted.

In several regions depleted groundwater, polluted water supplies, and competition from nonfarm users are reducing the agricultural water supply. Groundwater depletion is especially serious for irrigated agriculture. When groundwater is pumped faster than it is replenished, aquifers become depleted. It is estimated that nearly 10% of the irrigated area in the world depends on overpumped water. If overpumping continues, some crop areas will be lost from production entirely.

As urbanization expands, cities compete with farms for available water. In some countries, the choice has to be made between assuring the fresh water supply for cities or irrigating nearby farmlands. In the United States, ownership of farmland can carry with it irrigation water rights. This is particularly relevant in the Southwest where farmland would be virtually useless without access to precious irrigation rights. Towns or cities sometimes purchase or lease irrigation rights to assure adequate fresh water. This form of water triage usually favors urban dwellers and converts hundreds of thousands of acres of farmland into other uses.

Agricultural productivity can also be lost because water is polluted to the point of being unusable for irrigation. In coastal regions, as water tables are depleted, aquifers are vulnerable to invasion by seawater. This makes the aquifer no longer useful for irrigation, or any other fresh water purpose, for that matter. In Israel, for example, the main water supply for citrus growers is a coastal aquifer that has had a 50% increase in salt levels over the past 25 years. Moreover, about 10% of wells in that small country yield water that is too salty to be used on crops. India, Pakistan, Bangladesh, and China have the same problem, sitting over salty groundwater in major coastal regions. In India, millions of acres of farm land have been damaged by the use of salt water from a polluted coastal aquifer in Maharashtra, the state with a population of 100 million that has Mumbai as its capital and which requires an ever-expanding market basket to feed its rapidly growing population. Mumbai is destined to be at the top of the list of mega-cities by 2025, with more than 20 million inhabitants. Moreover, water pollution by industrial wastes is a serious problem. In China, the use of polluted water for irrigation is responsible for the loss of over 5 million tons of grain annually.

Around the world, adequate sources of water for agricultural expansion are simply not available. There are already several nations that use more than 100% of their annual renewable water supply by overpumping groundwater. This means that, sooner or later, their aquifers will be drained to a level of uselessness. As the population grows and aquifers are pressed harder to provide water for urban and irrigation purposes, the number of countries in this desperate situation will increase substantially by 2025. Most of these countries are in the Middle East and North Africa, where the struggles over water have already begun and are likely to intensify. Countries will have to reach agreements and sign treaties on sharing water to avoid the potential water wars of the new century.

One thinks immediately of the Euphrates and Tigris as rivers that have to be shared by political adversaries. But there are similar situations throughout the world. On the United States–Mexico border, Nogales, Arizona, and Nogales, Sonora, share the same aquifer as the main source of water for both communities. Upstream development in Mexico and rapidly growing water demands cause great concern for downstream users in Arizona, but efforts to reach agreements on groundwater use have been unsuccessful until now.

On the Indian subcontinent, there is also disagreement that leaves Bangladesh unprotected against unilateral action by India that could threaten Bangladesh's food security severely. The two countries share the vast Ganges-Brahmaputra river systems as they form the deltas that surround much of Bangladesh's habitable land before emptying into the Bay of Bengal. The Ganges passes through more than 100 Indian cities before reaching the estuary. Most of these expanding urban centers do not use treatment facilities before passing sewage into this holy river. In addition to urban sewage and the discharge from factories, the river carries the runoff from farmlands laden with chemical fertilizers and pesticides. Each country's actions concerning water use affects the other. River diversion in India resulting in reduction in the Ganges sediment load could lead to a rise in sea level in Bangladesh. Without cooperation on river control by the two neighbors, as much as 20% of Bangladesh's land could be under water by 2050. Agreements to manage these shared rivers have been the subject of frequent negotiations between the governments of India and Bangladesh. But time is running out. Each will double its population before 2050.

The Nile-dependent clusters of nations are among the world's fastest growing populations. Nine African countries share the waters of the Nile River basin with Egypt. More than 90% of the natural flow of the Nile is used for irrigation or is lost through evaporation. The water that reaches the Mediterranean Sea is heavily polluted with irrigation drainage and industrial and municipal wastes.

When President Abdul Gamal Nasser of Egypt decided to embark on what was to be in the 1950s the world's most ambitious dam project, he disregarded the advice of soil experts who saw the loss of precious topsoil as an unavoidable consequence of creating a huge lake of the Upper Nile valley. The Nile transports an average of 110 million tons of silt each year, much of it rich soil from the Ethiopian highlands. For thousands of years, 90% of this silt reached the coast to replenish the delta and the remaining 10% was deposited on the Nile floodplain, enriching the soil of the farmlands along its path. With financial support from the Soviet Union, his Cold War ally, Nasser embarked on the ambitious construction project. His speeches boasted of the additional agricultural production that would make Egypt the breadbasket for the Arab people. In the 10 years between 1960 and 1970 it took to build the Aswan Dam, Egypt's population grew from 26 million to 38 million, an increase of almost 50% that would consume the total additional agricultural gain of the newly irrigated lands and still leave Egypt in need of imported food.

The waters of the Nile are Egypt's lifeline. Every drop is needed to help feed the people and support industry, yet the new lake loses 10% into the atmosphere through evaporation from its surface. On the positive side, the Aswan Dam has spared Egypt from the uncertainties of droughts or floods that have caused suffering for millennia and has also provided an important source of hydroelectric power.

But the Aswan Dam has also created problems by preventing the flow of silt and topsoil and, because the delta is not replenished, salination has crept inward from the Mediterranean Sea. Until a few decades ago, population levels were such that upstream development scenarios in Africa posed little threat to Egypt's water security. With the population increases projected for the countries of the Nile basin in the twenty-first century, this will no longer be the case. There is the potential for conflict if negotiated agreements on river control and water sharing cannot be reached to satisfy the needs of all concerned.

Worldwide, dams collectively store up to 15% of the earth's annual renewable water supply. New construction of high dams to create additional reservoirs is one means to rescue irrigation agriculture. The huge investments required would be economically attractive if food prices rise, provided there is sufficient fresh water available to dam and store in reservoirs.

Construction of dams is not only a huge financial investment, but also has social costs as people are forced from their homes to make room for the dam, a reservoir, and its supporting infrastructure. Mexico City's neighboring communities put up a determined fight to prevent the creation of a reservoir that was absolutely essential to meet the city's growing water needs in the 1980s. Ultimately, the reservoir plan prevailed, and surrounding towns had to be relocated while the farmland was lost. The city is still growing and so is the need for more water. By 2025, Mexico City will require fresh water to serve the needs of 8 million more people.

For the Three Gorges Dam under construction in China, more than 1 million people are being relocated, frequently to worse conditions than they left. These poor, powerless people have no option but to accept their plight. The situation is common enough to have sparked the formation of an international public service law movement to attempt to protect the rights of people threatened by forced displacement because of dam projects.

China's Three Gorges Dam will not repeat some aspects of the Aswan Dan scenario. Because it is underway during a time when China has reduced its population growth rate, it will definitely increase the per-person grain production of the world's most populous country. The substantial expansion of grain fields promised by this mammoth project will expand the world's irrigated land somewhat in the years ahead. Moreover, in spite of the bleak statistics on loss of land for cultivation in most of the world's regions there is a glimmer of optimism that acreage under cultivation will expand and play a role in meeting future food production needs as farmers everywhere discover imaginative, productive uses for marginal or previously neglected lands. Crops that can survive in high–aluminum-content soil, for example, are being planted in land previously left fallow. Immense acreages in Brazil unsuitable for that country's traditional crops have proved to be productive for raising soybeans. A sobering fact, however, is that with intense farming, unless affordable nutrient replacements are provided, these marginal lands will rapidly lose their economic value and will, once again, be abandoned. I have learned from talking with agriculture scientists brought together by the Rockefeller Foundation for a conference in Bellagio, Italy, that in the inventory of scientific inputs that can increase crop yields and overall agricultural productivity, soil science can play a significant role and should not be overlooked.

Intensive farming can deplete soil nutrients and lead to land degradation, perhaps less visibly than parking lots or golf courses, but it poses a greater threat to aggregate size of croplands. This is part of the dynamics of population growth. The larger the number of people to be fed, the more intense the farming, and the greater the stress on the health of the land. Cropland fertility depends on the 12 or so inches of topsoil, rich in nutrients, many minerals, microbes, bugs, worms, and other components needed to provide a nurturing environment for plants. When the topsoil is depleted, it can only recover by being allowed to remain fallow for many years. Artificial fertilizer can replace part of what is needed for the health of soil, but this is a short-term fix that may delay but cannot prevent the ultimate loss of overfarmed, depleted land.

The rate of erosion of topsoil far exceeds the glacial pace at which it is replaced. In the poor regions where most of the world's population lives and where almost all the growth of the next 25 years will occur, soil erosion and poverty are inextricably linked as cause and effect. Put in terms of a chemical reaction, it is reversible; it goes in both directions. Poverty leads to erosion and erosion leads to poverty. The despair of the poor leaves little choice but to engage in overfarming, overgrazing, deforestation, and overharvesting of fuel wood. Poor people end up with poor land.

The food–water–population interaction is a conundrum that has no simple solution. Fresh water makes it possible to irrigate cropland to increase yields per acre. High-intensity use of fertilizer and pesticides, also essential elements of high-yield farming, contaminates water and reduces its availability for all purposes, including irrigation. As populations grow, the need for food increases, and the stress on land and water is magnified. Both land and water are finite resources so that the supply of each for growing food cannot expand indefinitely without new technological inputs.

During the past 50 years of unprecedented population growth, the yield increases of elite varieties of grains and other crops more than offset the shortage of new croplands and loss of established farm acreage's through erosion, contamination, or pressures of urbanization. As the world adds another 2.5 billion people in the next 30 years, it will take another boost from science to simply feed the newcomers at today's inadequate level of worldwide nutrition. But the challenge is even greater. As globalization helps large numbers of people throughout the world to climb the economic ladder, their diet expectations rise to menus rich in items higher on the food chain that are much less nutritionally efficient than the direct human consumption of grains. Live-stock, for example, consume seven calories of grain in their feed for every calorie in the favorite food of a steak lover.

There are excellent prospects for yet further increases in crop yields through biotechnology and gene modification of foodstuffs. These modifications could also reduce the need for fertilizers and pesticides and conserve on the use of irrigation water. Agro-industry may guide the direction of these advances to capture the bulk of their benefits. Alternatively, the new biotechnologies could result in tailoring crops to specific needs, a reduction in the use of inputs that farmers have to purchase, and fewer environmental problems. Scientific advances may also relieve the world's shortage of fresh water for irrigation. Desali-nation of aquifers or seawater is almost certain to become reality as procedures are developed that are energy efficient and are economically feasible.

Eradicating hunger will require more than technological break-throughs in production of foodstuffs. Poverty is at the root of the prob-lem. Social factors to reduce poverty such as advancing women's edu-cation and status, together with enhanced food availability per person, all serve to reduce malnutrition.

A world population growing toward 9–10 billion, as projected for the twenty-first century, will give Malthusian theory another chance to prove itself. It will also challenge modern science to show, once again, that the Cambridge economist-cleric overlooked the tremendous poten-tial of technological advances for increasing the world's food supply. But even if science succeeds again and meets the challenge of feeding the growing population of the next 25–30 years, the biotechnology and agro-ecology leaders of this achievement, like Borlaug and Chandler, will surely glance over their shoulders. At projected growth rates, the next billions are not far behind.

9

Globalization, Population, and the Changing Environment

Every species changes the environment in which it lives. That is part of nature. Tropical ants can build mounds of sand higher than a man. Burrowing ferrets can dig extensive underground tunnel systems, elephants can strip the bark off large trees or snap strong saplings, and the gentle panda can eat its weight in delicate bamboo shoots every day. A dominant species can destroy the very ecosystem on which its future depends. But only one species has found the power to change the environment of the entire earth and its atmosphere. I once heard Australian anthropologist Valerie Brown make this point in a Bellagio seminar by saying, "There's no place on earth that has been left unaffected by man." I thought she was exaggerating as I remembered pristine places I have seen all over the world. I recalled the beautiful golden sands of a hidden cove on a small Greek island that seemed as if no one had ever set eyes on it before. But as I listened, I realized that her point was more profound. She was talking about humankind's ability to diminish the earth's ozone cover by releasing chlorofluorocarbons into the air or to change the constitution of the atmosphere by massive

163

burning of fossil fuels. She meant the damming of large rivers that can alter the ecosystem of an entire continent, the polluting of lakes and streams that can carry death and destruction to plant and animal life hundreds of miles distant. If you add Chernobyl-like accidents or the destructive potential of unleashing nuclear weapons, I think she made her point.

The unprecedented growth in human numbers is having profound effects on our physical environment. Nearly all the population growth, almost 100 million a year, is in Asia, Africa, and Latin America, the world's poorest regions. At its current population growth rate of 2.4% per year, Africa, the world's poorest region, with a population of 790 million in 2000, will grow (in spite of the tragedy of AIDS) to 1.4 billion people by the year 2025 and will be home to 2 billion in 2050. People are leaving rural areas for the cities in greater numbers than ever before, straining the inadequate infrastructure, water resources, and waste disposal facilities. Conversely, some of the world's poorest people are moving into forests and fragile watersheds in search of land and livelihood. At the same time, in the rich countries, industrialization, urbanization, chemical-intensive farming methods, and wasteful consumption patterns contribute substantially to environmental degradation, both locally and globally.

People have a right to seek higher living standards for themselves and their families. This is both an understandable goal and a challenge. How can the living standards of four-fifths of the world's population improve and consumption levels rise without damaging the planet's environment? Some believe that science will come to our rescue with technological advances that will solve environmental problems, one after the other, as they become acute. I take little comfort, however, in knowing that these techno-enthusiasts are mostly economists and not scientists. The conclusion of a summit of National Academies of Sciences of 58 countries, meeting in New Delhi in 1994 was more sobering:

> As scientists cognizant of the history of scientific progress and aware of the potential of science for contributing to human welfare, it is our collective judgment that . . . it is not prudent to rely on science and technology alone to solve problems created by rapid population growth, wasteful resource consumption, and poverty.

Here is an example of the kind of problem challenging science and industry today. Between 1950 and 2000 the total number of passenger car registrations worldwide increased from 50 million to more than 700 million. In 1950 three-quarters of all registrations were in the United States, while in 2000 three-quarters of all vehicles were registered outside United States. This is because car and truck sales are booming in the world's developing regions. The big multinational companies have rushed to set up manufacturing in China, India, and Latin America where there are growing markets. Their advertising encourages the attitude that affluence means owning your own car. I was driving through Beijing with a Chinese friend and noticed a large billboard showing a happy young couple looking admiringly at a new model Japanese car. He translated the Chinese characters for me: "Public transportation is not cool! Buy your own car!"

The big automobile companies are savvy to economic trends. Today, China and India have more middle-class consumers than all of Western Europe combined. India, with a 200-million-strong middle class, is the largest consumer market in the developing world. The rest of the 1 billion Indians, many still living in the depths of poverty, are eager to move up the economic ladder to join them.

With two cars sitting in my garage (one fuel-efficient, the other a gas-guzzling clunker), I have no right to scold the growing middle class in China, India, or Brazil for aspiring to have a family car (or two). But, as the population grows and economic globalization brings larger numbers into the consumer economy, will the earth sustain another 1 billion internal combustion engines, consuming gas and oil and spewing carbon dioxide? Even now, before the next billion cars roll off the robotic assembly lines, globally one-third of world crude oil consumption and 14% of carbon dioxide emissions can be attributed to motor vehicles. In the United States the comparable figures are 50% of oil demand and 25% of released carbon dioxide. Once carbon dioxide is emitted, it becomes evenly distributed throughout the earth's atmosphere. So our addiction for owning cars affects everybody's atmosphere everywhere.

Next it will be our turn to live with the emissions of the countries that will soon surpass us in auto use and carbon dioxide emission. There may be a short-term solution. New car-owners may take to the hybrid car that consumes far less fossil fuel for miles traveled. That's what I intend to get when I junk the clunker. In Italy, with government subsidy, the Fiat Company is working on a hydrogen-burning auto they expect to have ready for the market in 2010.

A study released by the U.S. National Intelligence Council (NIC) in December 2000 concludes that by 2015 there will be a 50% increase in the demand for energy worldwide. In this short span of years Asia will replace North America as the leading energy-consuming region, accounting for more than half of the world's increase in demand. The NIC report concludes that total demand for oil will rise from roughly 75 million barrels per day in 2000 to more than 100 million barrels in 2015. The increase alone is almost as much as OPEC's current production. Natural gas usage will grow by more than 100%, mainly stemming from the tripling of consumption in Asia. According to the NIC, by 2015 little Persian Gulf oil will be directed to Western markets; three-quarters will go to Asia.

Meanwhile, there may be some increase in solar and wind-driven energy production, but these sources will remain minimal in comparison to total energy produced. In 1997 only 14% of the world's energy was produced by renewable sources—that is, wind, solar, geothermal, and biomass. Nuclear energy remains stuck by concerns about safety. Switzerland, with its Alpine rivers providing the world's highest proportion of energy generated by hydroelectric power plants, still needs to supplement supply with nuclear-powered facilities. Now ending a 10-year moratorium on the construction of additional nuclear generation facilities, the Swiss may soon resume construction as energy requirements rise with affluence in the small country with the world's highest GNP per capita. The careful Swiss have never had an accident at any of their nuclear power plants. It may not be a bad idea for the world to depend more on nuclear energy, provided the Swiss run all the plants. Otherwise, there is no evidence of new, revolutionary thoughts about energy sources that are feasible.

The burning of fossil fuels continues to drive globalization of the world's economy. When the World Bank keeps a record of country-by-country energy use, it measures in terms of "metric tons of oil equivalent." The more we need, the more we pump. The world is running a triple-blind experiment that has an unknown outcome. Oil-producing nations and companies are blind to any consideration other than the economics of supply and demand; leaders of oil-importing countries are blind to any concern other than assuring that the oil spigot stays open at a reasonable price; and the consumer is blind to the local and global environmental effects of our thirst for fossil fuels. The conventional wisdom seems to be why worry, when 80% of the world's available oil and 95% of the world's natural gas still remain in the ground, and we are getting more efficient all the time at extracting it.

World regions with the most rapid increase in energy demands are not improving or cleaning up their methods of burning it. When fossil fuels are burned, carbon dioxide is released into the atmosphere. Geoscientists have a written record of atmospheric carbon dioxide levels throughout the twentieth century. It has risen 30%. By measuring air bubbles trapped in ice cores, scientists can guarantee us that the current levels are higher than at any time in the past 420,000 years. Once in the atmosphere, the natural rate of removal of carbon or carbon dioxide is very slow. For all practical purposes, once it's there, it's there to stay. Computer jargon has now spilled over into other sciences. Instead of a billion tons, we talk about gigatons. Annual carbon emission globally from burning fossil fuel is described as 6 gigatons per year. No matter how you say it, 6 billion tons is a lot of carbon particles for the earth's atmosphere to absorb.

To appreciate the implications of this release of carbon into the atmosphere, you need to understand the most elementary principles of climate control on earth. The study of climate is a complex, sophisticated science. Following is a highly simplified explanation.

The earth's surface is warmed by sunlight, amplified by the earth's atmosphere being able to radiate back to earth the infrared component as it bounces off the surface. This radiation, or "natural greenhouse effect," can keep the earth's average temperature at about 60°F instead of below freezing as it would be if the earth were heated only by the direct rays of the sun. The component of the atmosphere most responsible for the greenhouse effect is water vapor. Carbon dioxide is, after water vapor, the second most important gas producing the earth's natural greenhouse effect.

The buildup of man-made greenhouse gases is unrelenting as population grows, affluence and consumption rises, and the demand for carbon-intense technology increases. Rising affluence has a long way to go in the world's poor countries. At the turn of the century, these countries, with 85% of the world's population, accounted for less than 20% of total world income.

In the United States, carbon dioxide emission exceeded 1.5 billion tons in 2000. Russia and the other newly independent nations of the former Soviet Union raised their emission level to 1 billion tons in 2000, compared to a fraction of that back in the Cold War days of

1950 when very little money or energy was devoted to individual consumption. This is when Nikita Khrushchev was bragging that the Soviet system was going to bury us economically. But the Russians had to wait for the burial of Khrushchev's system before being able to enjoy the rising affluence that contributes to most of the increase in energy consumption and carbon emission. I have to confess to a certain level of cynicism when I observed the way of life in the old Soviet Union and Eastern Europe. I always felt that what would bring down the Berlin Wall was not only a rush to freedom, but also a dash for Volkswagens and Jeeps.

Energy utilization and emission increases have been greatest in the developing countries with expanding economies and rapidly growing populations. China has increased its carbon dioxide emission 30-fold since 1950 and India, Brazil, Mexico, and Indonesia each has had roughly a 10-fold increase. An additional sevenfold increase is expected in these countries by 2050. Given population numbers, both India and China can be expected to continue having large increases in total energy consumption in the immediate future. Each of these countries has the potential to reach and exceed the total tonnage of carbon emitted by the United States, a race that global bystanders watch nervously. China will move to the top by 2015. India and Brazil will not be far behind.

Can the atmosphere, now absorbing 6 billion tons of carbon annually, withstand a doubling or tripling without having an effect on global climate? The answer is no. There definitely will be an increase in global average temperature, but there is uncertainty as to the extent. A range of a minimum of $1.5°$ to a frightening $5.8°C$ is estimated in the NIC report. The imprecision is due to uncertainty about the exact level of future emissions and uncertainty as to the sensitivity of the climate system to respond to increases in greenhouse gas concentration.

As a candidate during the election of 2000, President Bush claimed there was disagreement about global warming and that it needed more study. This attitude prevailed during his administration until June 2002, when the Bush administration sent a climate report to the United Nations detailing specific and far-reaching effects that global warming will inflict on the American environment. For the first time, the administration acknowledged that the burning of fossil fuels sends heat-trapping greenhouse gases into the atmosphere. The United Nations completed in 2001 a 1000-page report on climate change research conducted by 700 scientists. The report concludes that temperature rise is inevitable and that there is clear evidence that industrial pollution is to blame.

In a region-by-region breakdown, the U.N. report describes the impact that can be expected from global warming. In Africa, less water will be available and desertification will be worsened as average annual rainfall declines. Coastal settlements in many countries will be hit by rising sea levels, coastal erosion, and salination of coastal aquifers. The snows of Kilimanjaro, the seemingly indestructible ice cap made famous by Ernest Hemingway, may well disappear in the next 15 years, taking with it the natural irrigation system for the rich farmlands at its base. I spoke recently with a Tanzanian journalist who did a story on the melting of the ice cap of Kilimanjaro. She told me that when the snows are gone, the fertile lower hillsides and surrounding valley will dry out and become useless for farming unless they are irrigated in some way, a highly unlikely prospect considering the cost. When she explained this to the poor farmers who survive off that land, they could not be concerned about something that was 10 or 15 years off. What would alarm them would be if the factory in Arusha were forced to close for failing to meet carbon dioxide emission standards. Their sons work there and send home money.

In Asia, high temperatures, drought, floods, and soil degradation will likely diminish food production in arid and tropical regions. Northern areas may see an offsetting rise in productivity. Rises in sea level and more intense tropical cyclones could displace tens of millions of people in low-lying coastal areas of temperate and tropical Asia.

Southern Europe will become more prone to drought. In other areas, flood hazards will increase. Agricultural productivity may increase in northern Europe but decrease in southern Europe. Half of Alpine glaciers will disappear by the end of the twenty-first century. Latin American floods will become more frequent. Subsistence farming in northern Brazil could be threatened. Diseases such as malaria and cholera may increase. North America could benefit from modest warming, but there will be strong damaging effects in some regions. Rising sea levels could increase coastal erosion, flooding, and lead to more storm surges, particularly in Florida and on the East Coast. Diseases like dengue fever, malaria, and Lyme disease may expand their ranges in North America. Climate changes in the polar regions are expected to be among the largest anywhere. Already, the extent and thickness of Arctic Sea ice have decreased, and permafrost has thawed in Alaska and the Canadian tundra. The trends may continue and cause irreversible impact on ice sheets, global ocean circulation, and sea levels even long after gas emissions have been stabilized.

The NIC foreshadowed the U.N. report, predicting that during the next 15 years, "Global warming will challenge the international community as meltdowns of polar ice occur, sea-level rises, and the frequency of major storms increases." Any delay in international agreement to stabilize industrial emission levels will be costly in the long run and only increase the difficulty of finding solutions.

The need for continuing research notwithstanding, we certainly know enough to reach agreement on the Kyoto Protocol on Climate Change, an outcome of the 1992 Earth Summit in Rio de Janeiro. It calls for "stabilization of greenhouse gas concentrations in the atmosphere at a level that would prevent dangerous interference with the climate system." It can be done through cooperation between countries that can increase carbon sequestration by forest and other land conservation projects and countries that can undertake clean energy-development projects. For the industrialized nations, this will require a reduction in emissions before stabilization. The United States is called on to reduce emissions by 7% by 2008–2012. It will be too late if the presidents between now and then leave it to the man or woman who is inaugurated in 2008.

The argument that the protocol unfairly burdens the United States, which has less than 5% of the world's population and is responsible for almost 25% of the world's greenhouse gases emission, seems indefensible. If anything, the world has been living with the unfairness created by the appetite for fossil fuel in the United States and other industrialized countries. Undoubtedly, there are difficult issues to resolve in negotiating agreement. Countries with advanced systems for regulating, monitoring, and enforcing believe they will be penalized in an agreement with countries that are less likely to meet these requirements. But this is one negotiation that cannot be abandoned without agreement being reached.

The reason we should act now is that the possible consequences of not acting are too serious to risk. As I have described, the NIC and the U.N. reports warn that global warming of 1.5–5.8°C will have a wide range of adverse consequences, some of them irreversible and some of them unpredictable.

Ecosystems carefully balanced with precise physical characteristics will be particularly vulnerable. Sustained temperature elevations will lead to the extinction of many species. It is hard to quantify the loss when we change ecosystems in a way to destroy untold numbers of undiscovered species. How, for example, do you place a price tag on lost plants that may have had medicinal uses?

Climate change will critically worsen the shortage of water supplies in some regions and enhance flooding conditions elsewhere. While there can be solutions to water management problems, many of them would be long range and, for political reasons, not likely to be implemented. Politicians don't like programs with short-term sacrifices and long-term pay-offs, long after they are out of office. An admirable exception is South Africa's new democracy where the legislature has enacted the most progressive water policy in the world summed up in the motto, "Some for all, forever."

Sea-level rises can be expected because of both the temperature-related expansion of water volume (an experiment you probably did in high school chemistry) and an increase in the rate of melting of polar ice caps. As it happens, the world's coastal regions are where the global population is growing fastest. These will be the vulnerable areas, including Egypt's heavily populated Nile delta, or the string of offshore islands marking the inland channel of the eastern coast of North America, from the Florida Keys to Newfoundland. Small archipelagos like the Marshall Islands will disappear.

I remember the Marshalls from my service in the U.S. Navy. Beautiful places with enchanting names like Kwajalein, Enewetak, and Bikini, were hard to get a navigational fix on because they had elevations just a few feet above sea level. We knew nothing about global warming then, but speculated that the islands would disappear if ever struck by a typhoon-driven tidal wave. Instead, it was a man-driven calamity that struck Bikini on July 1, 1946. That was the time of the first U.S. atmospheric atomic bomb test over the Bikini atoll during Operation Crossroads. My ship was just over the horizon, out of sight of the island, on the morning when the B-29 Superfortress flew over the target area and dropped the weapon. It exploded into a gigantic fireball on the ocean's surface, followed by an awesome, pink mushroom cloud that rose up and up and then drifted off in a direction opposite from where APA 27 and our sister ships of Joint Task Force One were waiting. Although we didn't know a lot about atomic radiation, we wondered at the time if anyone might be downwind who hadn't been warned. As for us, we were back in the harbor that afternoon, feeling safe because of the routine clickings of handheld Geiger counters. I'd like to visit Bikini now that it has been declared inhabitable and the original families allowed to return. I wonder how they decided. Do you think it was handheld Geiger counters again?

With climate change, we can expect an increase in natural disasters. The 1990s set a record for losses from natural disasters caused by extreme weather events. In 1992, Hurricane Andrew left 250,000 people homeless in Florida and caused $25 billion in property damage. Central America has not recovered fully from Hurricane Mitch, which took 10,000 lives and brought untold misery in 1998. On Cape Cod, 1991's Hurricane Bob leveled pine forests and left us without power for 10 days, but we were spared loss of life. The unexpected nor'easter the following month, documented in print and film as *The Perfect Storm*, caused more damage and loss of life. As population density increases in coastal areas and more and more people are directly affected by these natural disasters, the cost in human lives and material loss can be expected to rise.

Geologists also worry about surprise events that are not now predictable but that may be triggered by climate changes of the magnitude forecasted. Changing temperature differentials could alter circulation patterns of ocean waters. This pattern of currents is vital to maintain the temperature norms of the North Atlantic regions of both Europe and North America. Even a minor but irreversible change could prove disastrous to agriculture and living conditions in the NATO countries. This could lead to mass migration in search of survivability. The NIC in its Global Trends 2015 report avoids the question of how global warming may affect political stability, but this effect might be the greatest threat to the security of Europe and North America.

The most effective action the world could take is to reduce the release of greenhouse gasses in the atmosphere and reach stabilization of the emission level. This is essential and is one of the objectives of the Kyoto Protocol. But there are other measures, as well, that are also included in the protocol. How we manage ecosystem resources that remove carbon dioxide from the atmosphere will have a significant impact on future increases or decreases. Large quantities of carbon dioxide are extracted from the atmosphere by the oceans, vegetation, and soil. Before man-made emissions became such an important factor, this exchange maintained relatively constant levels of the gas in the atmosphere for billions of years. Some ecosystems are more efficient in trapping and storing carbon dioxide than others. Forests and grasslands are good at removing and storing significant amounts of carbon, but agricultural land stores less. Land-use conversion from forests or grasslands to agriculture results in less vegetation per acre and creates a net loss in the capacity to store carbon.

The ocean and its flora is another huge sink for carbon dioxide. This makes the subject interesting to the scientists of Woods Hole, Massachusetts, home of two of the world's outstanding research institutions, the 113-year-old Marine Biological Laboratory and the Woods Hole Oceanographic Institution, whose research vessel, *Alvin*, discovered the resting place of the *Titantic*.

At the Marine Biological Laboratory an M.I.T. scientist recently gave a lecture explaining how scientists are exploring ways to increase ocean carbon dioxide sequestration by seeding large ocean expanses with iron to encourage the growth of certain plankton. Does it sound like heresy to suggest dumping the last billion cars on the ocean floor even as the next billion cars are ordered and ready for delivery? It may sound bizarre, but it could increase the carbon dioxide-carrying capacity of the oceans and create breeding grounds for ocean life to make up for the gradual loss of coral reefs caused by pollution and global climate change. This depends, of course, on the right type of plankton being stimulated by the iron.

Methane also contributes to the earth's natural greenhouse effect. Like carbon dioxide, this gas comes from both natural and man-made sources. Methane is a product of anaerobic metabolism. In nature, large quantities of methane are produced in wetlands and by farm animals that expel methane as a by-product of their digestive process. However, man-made sources are estimated to be about twice as large as natural sources and have led to more than a doubling of methane concentrations since record keeping began. This methane comes from leakage from natural gas pipelines and coal mines, anaerobic respiration in rice paddies, livestock raised for food or fiber, and biomass burning. Because it has a relatively short atmospheric lifetime, methane's effect on climate is shorter than that of carbon dioxide.

Man-made gas emission is an example of the importance of human behavior as well as human numbers. Americans have adopted a lifestyle that requires nearly 10 tons of oil equivalents for energy production and emission of 20 tons of carbon dioxide for every person each year. The Swiss, with an average GNP well above the U.S. average, live very well on less than half that amount of oil equivalents for energy and less than-one third the per-capita emission of carbon dioxide. Is it the French or Italian lifestyle you admire? They, too, manage on less than half the oil equivalents for energy production and less than one-third the emissions of the United States.

It is not just the earth's atmosphere that is changing. The earth itself, its resources, and the species that inhabit the globe are changing. Darwin taught us that there is always change going on: new species originate; species are lost. That's evolution. Even Kansas schoolchildren know that. But control over the rate at which species have been lost in the past century has been taken over by man-made activities everywhere. Deforestation, conversion of grasslands to agricultural use, and draining of wetlands have been primarily responsible for the loss of biodiversity. These are the disappearing ecosystems that are, by far, the richest source of the earth's plant life. Forest cover has been reduced by 20% worldwide. Some forest ecosystems, such as the dry tropical forests of Central America, are virtually gone. Wetland areas have shrunk and grasslands have been reduced by more than 90% in some areas. The U.S. National Research Council (2001) and the U.N.'s Food and Agriculture Organization place the annual tropical deforestation rate at about 40 million square acres. Of the estimated 4–5 million living species of plants and animals, about 3 million are found in the tropics, associated with forest cover. It is estimated that botanists have studied only about 10% of them. Yet, we are driving plant species from the earth faster than we can study their potential for medicine, food, or other uses beneficial to humans.

Regardless of broader ecological considerations, self-interest alone should give us pause. Plant species have played a major role in the development of foodstuffs and in treating ailments throughout history. The New York Botanical Garden keeps a collection of dried specimens of plants collected from around the world. Although more than 5000 of them are catalogued as being useful for food, medicine, aromatics, or dyes, few have been studied. Scientists from major pharmaceutical companies scan the globe for plant products that can hold clues to new chemical entities useful for human therapy. When we wipe out the plant species that scientists have never had a chance to evaluate, have we lost new treatments for cancer or heart disease?

In the early 1960s the National Cancer Institute funded a program to screen a wide variety of plants for biological activity. Out of that effort came the discovery that the bark of the Pacific yew tree (*Taxus brevilfolia*) had antitumor activity in laboratory animals. The mechanism of action of this compound was novel in the approaches to cancer therapy. It altered structures within the cancer cell in a way that made it impossible for cell division to take place. The active substance taken from the bark was named taxol, and it quickly proved to be effective for the treatment of drug-resistant breast cancer. However, isolation of taxol from the bark involves killing the rare tree, and the quantities recovered are pitifully small. It would take six 100-year-old trees to provide enough taxol to treat just one woman. This shortage and the novel mode of action prompted a search for a new class of cancer drugs that would be similar to taxol. Now chemists have worked out methods to totally synthesize taxol, and several taxol-like products are available for the treatment of breast, ovarian, and lung cancer.

Taxol is a story of the past few decades. The story of reserpine started hundreds of years ago. It is a plant substance obtained from the snakeroot plant, *Rauwolfia serpentina*, a small evergreen shrub native to tropical India. Known in India as *Sarpaganda*, it has been used for centuries in Ayurvedic medicine to treat fevers, snakebites, and other afflictions. In the 1950s, Western scientists isolated an alkaloid substance, named reserpine, from the plant, and it proved to be effective in reducing the risk of heart disease in people by lowering blood pressure. Like taxol, reserpine is now totally synthesized and in spite of a plethora of new products to control high blood pressure, it remains in the *Physician's Desk Reference* for treatment of hypertension.

I have a fond memory of *Rauwolfia serpentina* from my time in India serving as an advisor to the director of family planning, Colonel B. L. Raina. He assigned me the task of responding to questions from Parliament asking why India wasn't using Ayurvedic drugs instead of Western methods of birth control. Almost always, the question would start by reminding us of the *Rauwolfia serpentina* story. I set up a screening program in the laboratory to test the plant materials legislators would bring to New Delhi from their constituencies all over India, convinced these leaves or roots would be the answer to India's rapid population growth. With experience backed up by laboratory data, I became adept at convincing legislators that just because an Ayurvedic drug might relieve the symptoms of gout, for example, it didn't mean it would work as a contraceptive. I found that these skills came in handy later when called to testify before U.S. congressional committees. Once, after I had given testimony on governmentally sponsored research to develop new contraceptives, the committee chairman, a distinguished congressman from Wilkes Barre, Pennsylvania, who had been in his younger days a Shakespearian actor, leaned over his table and whispered to me, "Don't they use rubbers, anymore?" I assured him that research was continuing to improve the condom.

Rachel Carson's warning about chemical pollution seems to have had its 15 minutes of fame and then faded into obscurity. The amount of industrial pollution that has poisoned land, seas, streams, and lakes throughout the world since the publication of *The Silent Spring* in 1962 is shocking. When I learned recently that much of the research for her books on the sea was done at the Marine Biological Laboratory library in Woods Hole, I went back and reread some of her works. How could we have failed to pay attention? She was on to the danger of persistent organic toxins used as pesticides and for industrial purposes, yet the examples of continuing irresponsible dumpings is virtually endless: Love Canal in upper New York State; DDT disposal in the ocean off southern California; dioxins all over the world; trichloroethylene in Woburn, Massachusetts; chemical pollution in Russia and Ukraine; industrial disposal of mercury in Minamato Bay, Kyushu, Japan; pesticide runoff into most of the world's rivers and streams. Almost anyone you talk to can tell a story of a local pollution problem in their community. Rivers and other waterways have been particularly vulnerable and abused.

Running through the country's breadbasket, the Mississippi River suffers virtually uncontrolled pollution primarily because of agricultural runoff, but also because of the growing size of cities and towns along its banks. As it makes its long run to the delta, it is the source of the water supply and the basin for sewage disposal of town after town along the route. Each town is careful to take its drinking water from upstream and dump its sewage downstream of the community. It has always puzzled me why they bother doing this knowing that the neighboring town to the north is following the same logic.

Around the world, the fate of other great rivers is similar or even worse. For most of its length, the Ganges is an open sewer, and even its legendary cleansing power cannot save it. This once-majestic mother-river of India springs from glacial caves in the Himalayas, then flows east across the plains of northern India and down into the Indo-Bangladesh delta, where it empties into the Indian Ocean. Its river basin and delta support half a billion people, and this number is projected to rise to 750 million by 2020. Now, more than 100 cities and thousands of towns and villages extend along the banks of the Ganges. Because 80% of them have no sewage treatment facilities, wastes go directly into the river, along with thousands of animal carcasses. More pollution is added by hundreds of industrial sites. The factories of India manage to dump into their famous river just about every industrial toxin known. With population growth and added affluence in India, industrial discharge into the Ganges is increasing by 8% a year.

Unless India and its neighbors find a way to save this great waterway, the rivers of north India will not be able to provide a life-support system for the huge population of the Gangetic plains. India and Bangladesh need to give high priority to installing sewage treatment systems, not only along the Ganges, but also throughout their countries where similar conditions prevail.

It's the same throughout much of the world. The European Community passed a law in 2001 that will pave the way for a major cleanup of Europe's rivers and lakes and that bans industries from discharging hazardous substances into them. A key element of the directive is that it will require that neighboring countries that share the same river basin to work together to improve water quality in cross-border areas, preventing pollution from one country from damaging the environment in another country further downstream. Rachel Carson would be pleased.

The Nile is the longest river in the world. From its major source, Lake Victoria in east-central Africa, it flows north through Uganda and into Sudan, continuing to flow north into Egypt and on to the Mediterranean Sea. Ten countries with a population of 150 million make up the Nile River basin and are dependent on the river for their water needs. In just 20 years this number is likely to grow to nearly 300 million. Access to the waters of the Nile has already been defined as a vital national priority by both Egypt and Sudan. Each country has professed a willingness to go to war over it. As the countries of the Nile basin grow in population and improve their economies, the need for water in the region will increase. This is one of the world's hot spots where water wars may break out. Water withdrawal and river modification has so affected the natural flow of the Nile that it no longer reaches the Mediterranean during the dry season. The Aswan Dam has stopped the deposition of silt from the rich African soil so that the species dependent on the soil enrichment brought to the delta have disappeared. Indeed, the delta itself is disappearing. Instead, salination is creeping upward from the sea, making valuable aquifers unusable for irrigating farmlands.

Given the state of the world's rivers, it should be no surprise that the biodiversity of freshwater ecosystems around the globe is seriously threatened. More than 10,000 species, or 20% of the world's freshwater fish, have become extinct or threatened in recent decades. Exploitation, pollution, and the introduction of non-native species all contribute to declines in freshwater biodiversity. In Lake Victoria, when the commercially profitable Nile perch and tilapia were introduced, they overcame the native species to the point of extinction, a great tragedy for the local communities that depended on the native fish for food and did not benefit from the new ones.

Marine species have not fared better. Covering more than 70% of the earth's surface, the oceans are treated as huge dumping grounds for anything humans want to dispose of. The types of wastes that have been dumped in the oceans off the United States, for example, include acids, refinery wastes, paper mill wastes, pesticide wastes, garbage, explosives, radioactive wastes, and municipal sewage discharges. Commercial species such as Atlantic cod, some species of tuna, and haddock are threatened globally, along with several types of whales, seals, and sea turtles. Mercury contamination has given a new, unsettling, connotation to fish as a brain food. In the United States and some European countries, a growing number of fish types are being added to the list that could be too highly contaminated with mercury to be eaten safely by pregnant or nursing women. Mercury toxicity is of particular concern for the developing fetal brain, so that exposure in the womb can cause learning deficiencies for children. Popular fish such as swordfish and mackerel are already on the list, and some environmental groups believe that tuna, sea bass, and halibut should be added.

Overfishing also takes its toll. Jakob Jakobsson is an Icelandic scientist who should be considered an environmental hero. Studying the North Atlantic herring, the catch that supports the commercial fishing economy in Iceland, he realized in the 1970s that the schools of herring in Icelandic waters were disappearing. He undertook to persuade the fishing community to keep the fleet in port and give the herring two years to recover. It was financially hard on the families of herring fishermen, but because Jakobsson was from a family of generations of fishermen, they trusted him and followed his advice. The two-year moratorium saved the species and the small country's economy. Now, fishing takes are carefully monitored to prevent a similar situation from developing.

The environment is being changed both by how many people there are and what they do. America didn't need a population of 280 million to eliminate the bison from the Great Plains; we managed to bring it to the verge of extinction by the end of the nineteenth century with a mere 75 million inhabitants. Even one person can change the environment. When Eugene Scheifflin released 60 European starlings in New York's Central Park in 1890, he began a starling population multiplication that spread throughout the entire North American continent. At five eggs a breeding season, it doesn't take long, without natural predators, for an invader species to run amok. I had heard that account of the starling's entry into the United States but could never understand why Scheifflin, a wine importer, would be involved. I was enlightened when I met and became friends with his great-granddaughter, Olivia Scheifflin Nordberg. The family story, she told me, is that he was nostalgic for his native Germany after immigrating to the United States and thought it would be nice to have the familiar starling in his New York neighborhood as a reminder of the old country.

Aware of the starling story, I was concerned when, on a trip to Barbados, I met an elderly Englishman who was keeping a large, screen-enclosed aviary in which he was breeding tropical African birds with beautiful, colorful feathers. I recognized the birds because I had done research on the hormonal control of their feather coloration. The males, my studies proved, could grow the ostentatious nuptial adornment without the macho influence of testosterone. They used a different hormonal control mechanism. When my new friend explained that he planned to release the African weaver finches and Paradise wydahs when their numbers grew, I gently suggested that there are dangers in letting loose a foreign species in a balanced ecosystem. My knowledge of their scientific names and my account of why they had brilliant feather coloration didn't quite satisfy him of my ornithological expertise, so I urged him to contact the Audubon Society before going further with his plan. Some weeks later, I was delighted to receive a letter telling me that he had been sufficiently educated on the matter to give up his plan and that he would keep the birds enclosed for his own enjoyment.

Population pressure, overconsumption, and irresponsible human behavior exert threatening stresses and strains on the earth and its atmosphere. Anthropologist Brown had it right: There's no place on earth that has been unaffected by humans. The consequences can be anything from locally disruptive to globally disastrous. Shortages of fresh water, erosion of land, diminishing capacities of agriculture, and increases in the frequency of natural disasters are tribulations that affect everyone, but they pose a particular threat to the poor, who are already living on the edge throughout the world. Not infrequently, it is women who bear the brunt of family hardships and are left to find solutions to seemingly overwhelming problems.

The message of the 1994 Cairo population conference, the new paradigm, is clear: Empowering women is a component of fighting poverty and elevating the human condition. I believe that as women around the world gain more power, they will be leaders in their villages, cities, and countries in promoting environmental protection. Given a voice of authority, they will undertake to improve the circumstances of their own lives and to leave a better world for their children.

10

Reproductive Health, Education, and Gender Equality

International Women's Day is set aside each year to celebrate progress toward gender equality. In 2001 the first woman director-general of the World Health Organization marked the occasion at an event in Geneva. The former Prime Minister of Norway, a physician, bluntly declared, "There is not a single country in the world where men and women enjoy equal opportunity." Gro Harlem Brundtland's assessment is undeniable. She also noted the appalling fact that women in developing regions, particularly in Africa, die in pregnancy or childbirth at a rate 33 times higher than women in rich countries. This caught my attention because, as I mentioned in the introduction, it is a statistic that a previous director-general, also a Scandinavian physician, had labeled the most obscene of differences in health statistics. He was right then and she is right now. Between the two speeches, there has been a gap of 20 years. When will it change? Will another director-general 20 years from now be lamenting the same inequality? What is holding back progress? These tragedies of lives lost, children left motherless, and families ripped by despair are preventable with what we know now and with resources we have at our disposal.

The solution does not need to wait for advances or transfer of technology. It is a matter of setting priorities. Safe motherhood does not have sufficient priority in health care to receive adequate resources to back up the rhetoric. Pregnancy-related deaths occur at the rate of about 1 million a year, almost always in the poor countries, and most often in Africa and Asia. Women die because of obstructed labor, postpartum infection or hemorrhage, or botched and dirty abortions in places where politicians refuse to legalize the procedure so that women can have the choice and opportunity to have it done safely. Undetected toxemia of pregnancy also claims lives unnecessarily. These causes are all preventable and rarely take the lives of women in countries with adequate health care systems. With a minimum of good care most women will complete their pregnancies uneventfully; without it, women frequently suffer avoidable complications which can become life threatening.

As high as published maternal mortality rates are, because of underreporting the true figures are even higher. How do you suppose this death was recorded, for example? A friend was the chief obstetrician in a hospital in Egypt, along the Nile between Cairo and Luxor. This is a region of the country that showed early signs of fundamentalist influence. He told me of a young woman they saved when she came in with a raging infection after trying to self-induce an abortion following forced intercourse with a man in her village. Actually, the woman was raped. After days of intravenous antibiotics and surgical intervention, she pulled through. While she was recovering, her family came to her hospital room to visit. After they left, the hospital staff found her dead, smothered by her pillow. The case illustrates two causes of women's deaths that rarely show up in the reports on which national statistics are based: self-induced efforts to abort an unwanted pregnancy and so-called family honor killings that go unreported and unpunished.

The main causes of maternal mortality persist because health facilities in most poor countries do not assure the availability of essential services to all women during pregnancy and childbirth. Some countries like Nepal, Burundi, or Bangladesh allocate less than 1% of their public expenditure on health. Health-oriented countries like Sweden or Demark spend nearly 10% of their public expenditures on health care.

Simple measures can help without large financial outlay for capital equipment or construction, even in hard-to-reach regions like isolated mountain villages in Nepal. In these settings, women ready to deliver, without access to trained professionals, have to depend on the traditional birth attendant whose skills are passed down from mother to daughter. Their knowledge is rudimentary and, when complications arise, as can be expected in 10–15% of deliveries, they frequently can do more harm than good. But investing in the training of traditional birth attendants in simple procedures, such as clean cutting of the umbilical cord or promoting expulsion of a retained placenta by encouraging the newborn to suckle, can make a big difference in avoiding problems. In cultures where women cannot leave their huts or villages without permission from their husband, birthing centers staffed by trained midwives can serve as a substitute for a hospital or distant health clinic when a crisis occurs during delivery. Surveys in Malawi, for example, show that only 7% of men know that bleeding, fever, or long labor are signs that something is wrong. Yet in 70% of cases it is the husband who decides whether and when to seek help for his wife.

The concept of bypassing centralized health services and concentrating on training local people with minimal education to work in decentralized rural services is not new. In China a rural health program preexisted the revolution and communist government and continues today. I have visited many of these health centers in rural China and have always been impressed with some of their characteristics. Invariably, they are spotlessly clean, and the village-level workers ("barefoot doctors" of the communist years) proudly wear their white, cheflike starched hats. The villagers seem genuinely proud of their health station. Some villages I've seen were very poor, and I could imagine it must have taken some sacrifice to maintain the health station. China does not report the percentage of the population without access to health care. Nearby India reports that a quarter of a billion people still have no access to health services. Cuba is not a rich country and is tiny by comparison. Yet, by depending on rural centers, Cuba can report that none of its population is without access to health care. Cuba has one of the world's lowest maternal mortality rates.

There is plenty of blame to go around, but responsibility must begin with national governments that let their women and children die while finding money to spend for just about anything else. Huge mansions for the leaders, or a cathedral larger than Saint Peter's in Rome, to say nothing of amassed personal fortunes sitting in Swiss accounts, char-

acterize countries rich in natural resources but impoverished because
of the lack of investment in human resources.

How can one justify an average allocation of less than $6 per person
per year on all health expenditures in poor countries that spend small
fortunes to import weapons? Is it surprising that Burundi, which al-
locates 0.6% of its GDP to health care and spends 6.1% on military
expenditure, loses one child out of five from birth to five years old?
Relief organizations claim that in Afghanistan just one child out of four
survives until their fifth birthday. International organizations bear some
responsibility also. Official Development Assistance (ODA) to Burundi
in 2000 is a paltry $12 per person, a drop of 75% since 1990. Imag-
inative assistance programs, either to health ministries or through the
World Health Organization, could be directed specifically to safe motherhood.

There are also some worthy efforts that deserve recognition. The
World Bank's Health and Population Program took the lead 20 years
ago to focus world attention on maternal mortality. Leading the effort,
economist Barbara Herz found that the term "maternal mortality"
failed to generate much interest or enthusiasm, so she successfully lobbied to substitute the phrase "safe motherhood" as the theme for an
international conference in Nairobi. The Rockefeller Foundation and
other assistance agencies joined in, the term caught on, and the outcome after a successful Nairobi launching was an invigorated program
on safe motherhood at the World Health Organization in Geneva. The
new breed of super-rich philanthropists, including Ted Turner and Bill
Gates, deserve credit for focusing on women's health problems with
their mega-grants. Private foundations and charitable giving cannot
substitute for ongoing government commitment over the long haul, but
their demonstration programs can provide examples and save lives in
the process.

The risk of pregnancy-related death is the combination of the mortality rate per pregnancy and the number of times a woman goes
through a pregnancy. When both numbers are high, a woman's lifetime
risk is greatest. Reducing both is the best goal; reducing either is beneficial. From 1990 to 1998, the average American woman had 2 pregnancies in her lifetime, and the country's maternal mortality rate was
6 deaths per 100,000 live births. This means the chance of dying from
a pregnancy-related cause was about 1 in 8000. In Mozambique the
average number of children a woman has is 6, and the maternal mor-

tality rate is 1100 per 100,000 live births. For a Mozambique girl approaching adulthood, the chances of dying of a pregnancy-related cause is 1 in 15.

Throughout the world there is an unmet demand for contraceptive services and, consequently, a large number of unplanned, unwanted pregnancies. If all women could have the number of children they really want, the risk of maternity-related death would fall, infant and child mortality would decline, families would be smaller, and population growth would be slower. Moreover, if all women were given the level of education that the men in their families receive, they would marry at an older age and have fewer children. In addition, if women were provided with a package of reproductive health services incorporating family planning, safe motherhood, prevention and treatment of sexually transmitted diseases, and access to voluntary and safe abortion, deeply rooted injustices would begin to whither. And, if the reforms were extended to providing for universal education, to overcoming the bias of son preference, and to protection for female children so that they grow up safe, healthy, and equal, we could be on the way to a better life for the next generation.

Does this seem like a fantasy? Does it require high-powered technology? We could start achieving these goals tomorrow if we had the will. Countries must be willing to devote sufficient resources to make changes, starting with education. More schooling, especially for girls, is a fundamental investment in the next generation. Younger women, in particular, frequently are under coercive pressures to fulfill societal expectations with respect to marriage and fertility. The result is great pressure to marry early, have short intervals between births, and to have many children. In some societies, the husband and his family (the mother-in-law in particular) treat childless brides miserably even though a simple sperm count would reveal that male infertility is responsible about half the time. The longer the delay in first pregnancy, the greater is the maltreatment. It is not unheard of that childless young women lose their lives through "accidental" deaths at home, crimes that are simply left unpunished in these male-dominated cultures.

The distinguished Australian demographer, Jack Caldwell, said 20 years ago to expect a positive correlation between children's education and the overall measure of a nation's fertility and asserted that transition to low fertility in developing countries would be linked with the achievement of mass formal schooling. Experience has shown that he was right. The higher the level of education, the greater chance a woman has to take charge of her own life, and the fewer children she is likely to have. Ten years of schooling is correlated with a 50% drop in total fertility rate, compared to girls who are kept out of school. A positive correlation can be shown also between education and the percentage of couples using contraception. The poor countries of the developing regions of the world made great strides in education in the 1990s. Roughly 50 million more children were enrolled in primary school in 2000 than in 1990. Although the gap betweens boys and girls did not close and there are regional differences, this is a good start.

September 11, 2001, awakened New Yorkers, and the rest of the United States, to distant Afghanistan. Some years ago, I attended a luncheon meeting with State Department-sponsored leaders of the Afghanistan resistance that we were then supporting in their fight against the Soviet army. Then we called them mujahideen or freedom fighters. Now we know them as the deposed, ultra-fundamentalist Taliban. Clerically garbed and somber, the visitors spoke with confidence that they would create an Islamic state governed under the law of the Koran. One of them said that they would bring health care to the people and educate the children. I asked him if that meant they would educate the girls as well as the boys. He fixed me with a steely gaze and said, "We will follow the laws of the Koran." I'm no student of the Koran, but I'm willing to wager there is nothing in its teachings that calls for depriving young girls of education. The Taliban-imposed restrictions suffered by Afghan women were one of the world's great injustices of recent years. When the Taliban fell, a veil of oppression was lifted from the women of Afghanistan.

The continuing lack of universal school enrollment in India and the gender gap is in sharp contrast to China, where primary school enrollment is reported to be 99.8%. I mentioned in the introduction my disappointment that a project on this subject never got started during my years at the Rockefeller Foundation. V. Ramchandran, an economist at the Indian Embassy in Washington, D.C, proposed the plan. The idea was to demonstrate the value at the local level of keeping young girls in school. An input of external cash would benefit the family and the community, and the girls would get an education. It was not to be a bribe but a payment to offset the family's lost labor cost of sending the girls to school. Three villages were selected near the small city of Gwalior, in the state of Madya Pradesh, not far from Agra and its incomparable Taj Mahal. Ramchandran understood the culture of North India, so the proposal was that the small monthly payments for every year daughters were allowed to continue schooling would be paid to the fathers. He believed it would be unacceptable for the little girls or their mothers to receive cash payments directly or into accounts in their names. Moreover, including the lowest-caste families in the villages would have been impossible without the participation of the male Harijan leaders. When the proposal came up for funding, feminist colleagues argued that such a scheme would serve to maintain patriarchal dominance and the proposal was tabled. I regret that I did not insist that we give the plan a chance to prove itself.

Although human behavior is steeped in tradition and guided by culture, people recognize opportunities that are in their self-interest and respond rapidly to adopt new, beneficial modes of behavior. The fathers of Gwalior may very well have been able to live with the idea that extra spending money could come through the woman, not the man in the family. Subsequently, other assistance agencies and countries have moved the idea forward. Mexico has a program paying parents to send children to school. The grants increase for higher grades and pay more for girls than for boys. The use of public resources to subsidize girls' education has also been shown to pay off in Bangladesh, and Pakistan. "Knowledge is jewelry for girls that remains with them throughout their life. . . . I think knowledge is better than a dowry," was the reaction expressed by one Pakistani mother. So, this would be my advice: Enroll all children, particularly girls, in primary school and keep them there. Eliminate the gender gap in primary and secondary schools. This does not mean that government programs to provide family planning services are not necessary. If a woman doesn't want to become pregnant, there are only two options, abstinence or contraception, whether or not she can read and write. If you are literate but poor, government help with family planning is high on the priority list of what is expected from social services.

HIV/AIDS has become a women's reproductive health problem of enormous magnitude. Seventy-five percent of new cases each year are infections transmitted to women through heterosexual intercourse, most commonly because a husband, companion, or forced sex partner is sero-positive for HIV. Commercial sex workers are at high risk of acquiring AIDS and passing it on. AIDS victims are not only the young adults who become debilitated and then die, but also the children left without parents. In Africa, there are so many orphans as a result of AIDS that the burden is too great for surviving relatives to cope with. The problem has already spilled into the streets of African cities and elsewhere, where homeless street children abound. The magnitude of this problem is staggering. In Zambia alone the disease has created 500,000 orphans and in Uganda slightly more than 10% of all children under 15 years have lost one or both parents. AIDS has orphaned 12 million African children, and more will need care in the coming years.

A Centers for Disease Control epidemiologist, Dr. Kevin Decock, who works in Africa has written that, based on his experience with the AIDS epidemic on that continent, it is "a major public health emergency the likes of which the world has never seen before." He has called it "Africa's biggest issue since slavery." These statements are not exaggerations. The full scope of the disaster is beginning to be realized after decades of denial and inadequate response. Experts estimate that 20% of the adult population of several countries, including South Africa, is infected with the virus. It will be higher before the epidemic is checked.

The poverty and powerlessness of women make them increasingly vulnerable to AIDS. In many disadvantaged societies, girls and women do not have the power to reject unwanted or unsafe sex. In some parts of India, the myth has spread that a man can be cured of AIDS if he has sex with a virgin. Those HIV-positive men who can afford it buy the services of young girls, the younger the better to assure they are virgins, whose parents are too poor to turn down a cash offer that could feed the entire family for a month or a year.

The development of methods that a woman can use to protect herself against infection, without requiring male cooperation, deserves high priority. The only contraceptive method proven to reduce susceptibility to HIV is the condom, and its use depends on the willingness of the male partner. African men are beginning to overcome their reluctance to use condoms as they see it as a way to protect themselves against infection, but condom rejection is still high. There is little women can do to insist upon or negotiate its use. In fact, the practice of "dry sex" still prevails even though the resultant vaginal abrasions increase the chance of transfection in either direction. Men pay higher prices to commercial sex workers for dry sex, which involves clearing the vagina of naturally lubricating secretions for the purpose of enhancing the man's sexual pleasure.

Because it is sexually transmitted, AIDS prevention, treatment, and counseling have become essential elements of comprehensive reproductive health care. Vaccines are in the research pipeline but appear to be years away. Drug therapy is complicated and costly. Multiple drug treatments involving anti-retroviral drugs and protease inhibitors do not offer a cure, but they can slow down the progression of the disease and keep people alive longer. The truth is that the tens of millions of infected women and men in the poor countries of the world will die of AIDS as young adults. In richer countries, drug therapy can hold off the ravages of the disease longer. The preventive tools are straightforward but not that simple to introduce: abstinence or condom use, no multiple sex partners for either men or women, and antiviral drug treatment (such as AZT) for HIV-positive women who are pregnant.

New drugs are under study that may add to the array now available, but all are extremely expensive. Treatment for one patient in the United States can cost $20,000 a year. Even drastic price slashing is not likely to be helpful in countries that spend $6 per person on health care, the average in Africa's poorest countries. When I mentioned this figure recently to a health ministry financial official from strife-ridden Rwanda, she shook her head and told me that in Rwanda the annual per-capita money spent for health is $1.40. Conversing with us at the time was the finance minister from a neighboring African country. It was not reassuring that he had no idea what the per capita health budget is in his country.

Condom use and modification of sexual behavior can hold back the spread of AIDS. After being particularly hard hit by the epidemic, Uganda has demonstrated that a strong program based on this approach can be effective, and the country has halted the increase in annual infection rate. Senegal has also had success in curbing infection rate. In other countries the infection rate is increasing rapidly.

Early in the epidemic, I visited a friend who was the vice-chancellor of Kenyatta University in Nairobi, and we spoke about controlling the spread of AIDS. He told me that his young students viewed with skepticism the information they received on the risk of sexual transmission of HIV. They see it as scare tactics by authorities to control their customary sexual promiscuity. After the AIDS epidemic was recognized, the rite of sexual passage was still being practiced by upper classmen bringing prostitutes onto the campus to service the sixteen- or seventeen-year-old freshmen. Nairobi prostitutes by that time had an

85% rate of HIV infection, and both the vice-chancellor and I doubted that freshman week at the university brought on a surge in condom sales.

The disease crosses all social stratifications, from college students to truck drivers. One of my African friends, an obstetrician exposed to untested blood almost daily doing deliveries, lost his life to AIDS. In his case, living in Zimbabwe where more than 40% of pregnant women test positive for HIV was an occupational hazard.

Violence against women takes many forms and is often justified by cultural reasons. The culture plea has been offered to justify female genital mutilation, sometimes referred to using the euphemistic term "female circumcision." The actual procedure is brutal mutilation done for the purpose of depriving women of the clitoris and genital labia and in some cases to sew closed most of the vaginal opening to assure a future husband that he will be marrying a virgin or to remove the temptation for women to seek sexual enjoyment. This brutality not only leaves deep physical and psychological scars, it frequently results in reproductive tract infections that rob women of their fertility, carrying them into a life of misery that is the fate of sterile women in societies that value women according to their reproductive success.

A Sudanese woman physician I know, an ardent opponent of female genital mutilation, claimed that American feminists do not understand the cultural basis for this practice, so they should stay out of the fight. Fortunately, the international community does not hold her view. The Cairo agenda calls for governments and communities to take urgent steps to stop female genital mutilation and protect women and girls from all such similar practices. It calls for extensive education programs and appropriate treatment for girls and women who have suffered mutilation. Since 1995, twelve countries have adopted legal or administrative measures making female genital mutilation a crime.

Dr. John Kelley does medical missionary work in Tanzania as a gynecological surgeon. He has tried to help thousands of women by doing restorative surgery to correct the ravages of earlier genital mutilation procedures. Another admirable physician, Dr. George Povey, does similar noble work in Mozambique. These gynecologists also correct fistula formation between the bladder and vagina resulting from inadequate obstetrical care and frequent pregnancies. The constant leakage of urine creates a life of misery and isolation. In my opinion, this neglect is another form of violence toward women.

Throughout the world, unjust social structures and discriminatory attitudes deprive women of the opportunity to fulfill their potential and achieve their aspirations. Son preference results in higher rates of mortality among young girls, contrary to their genetic endowment for greater durability than boys. Sex-selective abortion deprives them of life.

When I was teaching reproductive medicine at the All India Institute of Medical Sciences in New Delhi, a new procedure was developed in Western medicine to differentiate between XX female cells and XY male cells, using a smear of exfoliated cells collected with a cotton swab from the inner cheek. It was based on identifying the condensed DNA of the second X chromosome, which could be visualized by special staining procedures. Absent from male cells, it is known as the Barr body, named after the Canadian doctor who first described it. With the aid of geneticist Dr. Harold Klinger, from Albert Einstein Medical Center in New York, we taught this procedure to young Indian gynecologists for its general usefulness in reproductive biomedicine. It could help, for example, in clarifying a diagnosis in cases of intersexuality or infertility.

During a visit to Bombay several years later, I met one of the students from that course. She shamelessly informed me how useful the technique was to determine fetal sex for couples requesting selective termination of a female fetus. I was angered to learn that, unintentionally, I had played an indirect role in this sexist behavior. Later, when I described how upset I was about this to a woman I admire greatly for her fight for women's reproductive rights and freedom, she pointed out to me that if you believe in choice, you can't impose limits for someone else. Either you believe in a woman's right to control decisions about her own body, or you don't. Nonetheless, I can't go along with sex-selective abortion. Maybe the answer is to widen women's education on this matter and give them more decision-making power within the family, so that they will abandon old ideas about son preference.

Many of the things I've written about seem so irrational as to be unbelievable. A husband who doesn't know anything about childbirth decides when his wife in labor needs to seek help, a young girl's sexual availability being sold by her parents to HIV-positive men; a woman is murdered for having disgraced the family by having been raped. If these were just anecdotal reports of isolated incidents, I could be accused of tabloid journalism, but these are patterns of behavior that affect hundreds of millions of women in their everyday lives.

I hope this chapter helps you understand why women's empowerment, education, and equality with men are vital issues in their own right, even if the proven impact on fertility reduction did not exist. Why has it taken us so long to move these issues to the top of the world's agenda?

11

Population and the Changing Burden of Illness

The burden of illness is changing as the age structure of the world's population changes. The average age is increasing as health improves for a greater proportion of people. The shifting composition of the less developed countries, where most of the world's people live, will account for most of the changing age structure over the coming decade, but the shift will be particularly prominent in the industrialized nations. By 2010, nearly 1 out of 4 people in Japan will be over 65. The countries of Western Europe will have 20% over 65, and in the United States, the proportion will be almost 15%. This means that health care needs will be gradually shifting into the circumstances of aging—more women in the postmenopausal years, more men with prostate disease, and for men and women a greater incidence of heart disease.

Age distribution is contributory, but the variables that most affect the disease status of people are population-related factors such as urbanization, slum dwelling, and air or environmental pollution. The relationship between these population-driven causal factors and health is striking and they can influence the health of rich and poor, rural and urban, and people of all ages.

Health risks imposed by conditions affected by population numbers and human behavior can be readily quantified. Animal models make it possible to test for toxic levels of pollutants, and scientists can use epidemiological and clinical studies to assess the health impacts on humans of exposure to noxious agents. Clinical studies involve laboratory tests and physical examination of people who have been exposed to the suspected health risk. There are different types of epidemiological studies but, generally, these are population-based studies that compare one group of people with another after one of the groups has been exposed to a potential health risk and the other has not. Data from these studies are essential because unsubstantiated assertions tend to weaken an argument and engender skepticism. Like Gresham's law, bad data tend to drive out good data. I recall a roundtable discussion at Columbia University. As I waited my turn to talk about population, I listened as other speakers discussed environmental issues. I suddenly realized that I had heard several times that "Breathing the air of New York City is like smoking two packs of cigarettes a day." I couldn't figure out how you would do the experiment to prove this, so I finally asked and the answer essentially was "Everybody knows that!" I didn't and I still don't believe they could prove it.

Based on quantifiable measures of air quality and other factors, urbanization may be the most important issue influencing the future health of global population. Massive and unprecedented migrations of populations from rural areas in the past few decades are fueling urban growth worldwide. As I discussed in an earlier chapter, even in the poorer, traditionally agrarian countries, more people now live in expanding urban and industrialized zones than at any time in history. In the 1950s New York was the only city area in the world with a population greater than 10 million. As the twentieth century came to an end, more than 20 cities were of that size or greater, and 18 of them are in the developing world. And there is much growth ahead. Mumbai had less than 3 million in 1950, 17 million in 2000, and will have 27 million in 2015. Jakarta is moving from 9 million at the turn of the century to an expected 21 million in 2015.

Poorly controlled industrial emissions and vehicular exhausts, causing high levels of air pollution, often accompany urban expansion. As families leave rural areas and flock to the cities, the widespread exposure of children to heavily polluted air is a mounting public health issue. Childhood asthma is reaching epidemic proportion. Developing countries are home to 85% of all the world's children under the age of 15, and roughly half of them live in cities where they regularly breathe dirty air. Consequently, exposure to pollution is a health risk to almost half the world's children, and the chances are that pollutant levels will continue to rise during their childhood.

Sam Keeney dedicated his life to helping the world's children. He was UNICEF regional director in Asia at a time when that relief organization saved millions of the continent's children from starvation. This was one of the achievements for which UNICEF received the 1965 Nobel Peace Prize. Keeney began his remarkable career when he left Oxford University, where he was a Rhodes Scholar during the First World War, to volunteer as an ambulance driver. He stayed in Europe to help with the postwar refugee problems, continued his humanitarian efforts in the years leading up to World War II, worked with Fiorello LaGuardia after the war in the United Nations Relief and Rehabilitation Administration looking after displaced persons, then went to UNICEF and finally joined the Population Council before bringing an end to his long and illustrious career. Beyond 90 years of age, Keeney made a final trip to his beloved Southeast Asia, where we gathered to attend a conference honoring him. He not only traveled to the conference, but also made a brilliant speech reminding us of the continuing need to protect the world's children. In Keeney's autobiography, *Half the World's Children*, he describes his efforts to help feed the world's impoverished children. Now, in addition to malnutrition, half the world's children of the twenty-first century face a new threat to their health brought on by the environmental pollution of the urban lifestyle they are born into.

Pollutants in the air can be scientifically measured, determining the precise health effects of these pollutants is more difficult, but objective information serves as benchmarks. The World Health Organization and other national and international groups have established guidelines for determining whether pollutants are exceeding acceptable limits. Three commonly measured pollutants are total suspended particulates, nitrogen dioxide, and sulfur dioxide. Extremely fine air particulates, whether they be asbestos particles or weapon-grade anthrax spores, cannot be seen but are most hazardous to human health because they are inhaled deeply into the lungs. In the weeks after the destruction of the World Trade Center, New Yorkers living in lower Manhattan had to contend with an enormous concentration of suspended particles in the air. The dean of Columbia University's School of Public Health, Dr. Allan Rosenfield, alerted the city's health facilities to expect an increase in respiratory complaints, and his prediction was borne out almost immediately.

Sulfur dioxide in the air brings contributes to a worsening of asthma and other lung diseases by causing constriction of the bronchial airways. Nitrogen dioxide tends to be high in regions where traffic density is high. This pollutant's effects on health include damage to the cells lining the bronchial tubes and lungs so that defense against microorganisms is weakened, increasing susceptibility to respiratory infections.

Air pollution generally affects children more severely than adults. A child's lung grows most rapidly during the first two years of life and continues to grow until the late teen years. This is a period of greater vulnerability than after physiological maturity has been achieved. Because they breathe at a faster rate, children also tend to absorb pollutants more readily than adults, and they retain pollutants in the body for longer periods of time. With growing affluence likely to bring a billion new vehicles to the poorer countries in the coming decades, air pollution in the developing world will worsen. Air pollution is already responsible for at least 50 million cases of chronic cough in those under age 14, according to the World Health Organization.

Study of infant deaths in the first month of life shows that those living in areas with greater air pollution exposure caused by small-sized particulate matter have a 45% higher risk of dying from respiratory illness than infants living in less polluted areas. In developing countries, many urban children are in double jeopardy from environment hazards and poverty. They live in polluted and degraded environments, and a significant number suffer from malnutrition and infectious or parasitic diseases.

The burden of illness caused by environmental pollution adds to the health effects of food deprivation, microbial diseases, and lack of preventive care or medical treatment. Children with diets deficient in vitamins, minerals, and proteins are especially vulnerable to toxic effects of chemicals. In the extreme case of acute chemical poisoning at the Bhopal tragedy in India, it was the children and elderly who were the most vulnerable. Children were also the victims of Chernobyl. At first, experts breathed a sigh of relief when there was no apparent increase in cancers after the nuclear plant meltdown in the Soviet Ukraine. After a few years, however, doctors began to encounter a growing number of thyroid cancers in small children. This was because radioactive iodine had been produced in the fallout, and the growing thyroids of both fetuses and infants had absorbed the cancer-causing isotope. Adult thyroids were unaffected because they already had reached maturity and were not absorbing external iodine in significant amounts. At the time of the accident, the simple administration of potassium iodide tablets to pregnant women and children would have saturated their iodine intake capacity and kept out the carcinogenic isotope.

Unfortunately, the tragedy of the AIDS epidemic has made immunodeficiency a household word. Less familiar is the possibility that certain chemicals in the environment can cause immunodeficiency. Many pesticides and other chemicals have long been banned or restricted in the United States, but these hazardous substances are still sold in large volume in developing country markets. DDT, chlordane, and parathion are examples from a list of more than 20 U.S.-banned pesticides that are still sold in other parts of the world. Many of the chemicals and the containers they are sold in litter rural farmlands almost everywhere. A Kenyan study found that cooking pots or water containers are used to mix pesticides which are stored in open containers in sleeping or cooking areas. Agricultural pesticides have even been used to eliminate head lice on children.

Warnings about the dangers of these chemicals, are often ignored. Global pesticide sales for use in agriculture have increased by more than 10% annually since the 1960s. That brings about a doubling every 7 years. The increase has been highest in poorer countries, eager to increase food production in order to avoid expensive imports. In Latin America use has tripled between 1980 and 2000. Sales by multinational agrochemical companies in developing countries are a multibillion dollar industry. In addition, many countries manufacture these products domestically.

Once when I was preparing for a trip to China, Edouard Sakiz, president of Rousell UCLAF of Paris, asked me if I would take along brochures describing a new agrochemical his company was marketing in Europe to replace more toxic substances. I did and left them with the appropriate agriculture ministry personnel in Beijing. Sakiz later told me that his company had subsequently set up a joint venture manufacturing facility in the rapidly decentralizing Chinese economy, and they were producing more of the product in China than for all the European countries combined. I take some satisfaction in believing that my intervention may have resulted in the replacement of more toxic substances.

Many organic and inorganic pesticides can pass from mother to fetus through the placenta or through breast milk, potentially leading to birth defects or retarded development of the immune system. Pesticides can also be consumed in food products because many of them do not degrade rapidly. Decades after DDT was banned in the United States, people who eat large amounts of fish from the highly polluted Great Lakes are likely to have DDT levels in their bodies twice as high as people who do not eat lake fish.

With urbanization and the widespread movements of displaced persons or refugees, drug-resistant tuberculosis (TB) is spreading and growing more dangerous. Untreated TB spreads quickly in crowded refugee camps. As many as 50% of the world's refugees may be infected with TB. The movement of displaced persons, the absence of health services in urban slums, and the emergence of multidrug-resistant TB are all contributing to the worsening of the global threat of this disease. Tuberculosis kills about 2 million people each year. The biggest burden of the disease is in Southeast Asia, but new outbreaks have occurred in Eastern Europe, where TB deaths are increasing after almost 40 years of steady decline.

The United States is far from TB-free. Countrywide, there were 18,000 new cases reported as recently as 1998. The disease is widespread in the prison population and among the homeless in large cities. Approximately 30% of San Francisco's homeless were infected with TB in 1995. Perhaps the biggest factor in the spread of TB in the United States is our openness in accepting immigrants from around the world 40% of TB cases are among foreign-born people.

Slum dwelling breeds tuberculosis as well as other diseases thought to have been eradicated or in decline. Along with the rapid population growth taking place in urban centers, there is a concomitant disproportionate growth in the number of slum dwellers. In some cities in the developing world, up to 70% of the population lives in slums. Drinking water sanitation tends to be poor. Standing pools of stagnant water make ideal breeding places for disease vectors such as the mosquitoes that carry Dengue fever or malaria. Garbage and disease-carrying rodents are everywhere, and there is a virtual breakdown in municipal health services in these slums. A study in Nairobi shows that slum living fosters risky sexual behavior and exposes young women, in particular, to increased risk of sexually transmitted diseases, including HIV/AIDS.

Mexico City's population will jump to nearly 20 million in less than 15 years. Dengue fever is emerging there and in other big cities of the Caribbean and tropical America, although it was virtually gone from the Western Hemisphere 20 years ago. Now, facilitated by breeding sites for the mosquito vector (*Aedes aegypti*) created by slum conditions, it has returned to Central America and the Caribbean, Venezuela, and the other Amazonian countries. Although dengue starts out as non-fatal, the more infections a person experiences, the more likely the disease will convert to dengue hemorrhagic fever, which is deadly. Dengue is not a tropical disease you are exposed to on jungle or mountain treks. You can catch it when you visit tropical urban areas, particularly if they are slums. The mosquito vector *Aedes aegypti* is both airborne and ocean going. It moves from city to city on tramp steamers carrying shiploads of discarded auto tires harboring pools of stagnant water and mosquito larvae.

Malaria remains a major health problem for tropical populations. It kills more than 1 million people a year, and its debilitating effect on families leaves them almost helpless to improve their circumstances. Increased risk of the disease is linked to human activities like mining, dam construction, and irrigation. International travel is carrying the disease back to areas where it was previously under control, and the emergence of multidrug-resistant strains is making the situation worse. The phenomenon of "airport malaria," or the importing of malaria by international travelers is becoming commonplace. Every day malaria victims from Africa land at Heathrow airport in London.

Malaria remains, however, primarily a disease of Africa. More than 90% of all cases are in sub-Saharan Africa. African children under five years of age often contract chronic malaria, which drains the vitality from those who survive. Throughout the African continent, the mass movement of refugees, displaced by political upheavals and economic necessity, is redistributing malaria and introducing it more and more from the countryside into urban centers.

Conventional wisdom is that because of its environmental risks, DDT spraying for mosquito control should be confined to interior house-by-house coverage in high-risk areas. DDT is hazardous to certain wildlife species, so that outdoor spraying is considered to be inappropriate. There is debate as to whether DDT is directly harmful to the health of people. It is an organochlorine that accumulates in the bodies of chronically exposed people. Significantly elevated levels can be found in the blood serum of people living in DDT-treated households. Some pesticides belonging to the same class of halogenated hydrocarbons are known have effects on the immune system of experimental animals. It seems logical that even without direct evidence of a toxic effect, DDT should be carefully handled to avoid unnecessary exposure of humans. Yet, there is no evidence-based verdict that DDT is harmful to people. Without such evidence, it is hard to dispute the conclusion of the distinguished physician and essayist, Gerald Weissmann, that banning the use of DDT has caused more deaths than HIV/ AIDS.

There have been several new drug therapies for malaria introduced in the past 20 years, but with multidrug-resistant strains to cope with, more new drugs are badly needed. You've probably heard that the British taste for gin and tonic goes back to the days of the British Raj in India, when quinine water was popular for fending off malaria. Quinine pills were also a required daily ration for American troops serving in the South Pacific. More recently, chloroquine was the drug of choice for many years, but there are growing areas of chloroquine-resistant malaria, so newer drugs such as proguanil, mefloquine, and doxycycline are available and new drug combinations are under investigation. An effective malaria vaccine is still 10–15 years away.

When he won the Nobel Prize in Medicine in 1958 at age 33, Josh Lederberg was the youngest person ever to receive that honor. I think he is the first person from whom I heard the phrase "newly emerging infectious diseases" long before it became a popular theme for novels, movies, and newspaper articles. Lederberg pointed out that viruses are humanity's only real competitors for global dominance and that we are currently not scientifically prepared to meet the challenges of potential viral outbreaks or transformation of present viruses into more deadly mutations. He is not alone in these concerns. D. A. Henderson, one of the leaders in the conquest of smallpox, believes that we have had ill-founded complacency about infectious diseases, trusting that antibiotics provide our safety net, but that we should realize that human health and survival will be challenged always with unpredictable infectious agents.

Time and evolution do not stand still. The human species is in a constant Darwinian struggle. Microbial and viral adversaries are in no less abundance than before, and they still present a constant threat to individual survival, as well as to large segments of the population. The plague wiped out one-quarter of the population of Europe in the fourteenth century. I believe our current rapid communications, scientific capabilities, and general state of societal organization protect us from so major a global epidemic catastrophe. Nevertheless, we must devote more of our national resources to strengthening even further our scientific and public health capabilities. According to the American Society for Microbiology, our public health system is not prepared to meet the challenges of new and reemerging infections or the threat of bioterrorism. We learned that soon after a few anthrax cases appeared in Florida, New York, and Washington, D.C.

Perhaps the most obvious defect is inadequate disease surveillance and reporting. The earlier the public health system knows what we are facing, the better the chances of combating it. As population centers become more numerous, the outbreaks of new or old infectious epidemics can only be more costly in terms of human lives and suffering. By the time a new pathogen is detected and a strategy developed for its containment, it may have already infected large numbers of people. To prevent the rapid acceleration of an epidemic, time is everything.

We need to spend hundreds of millions of dollars more than we now apportion to research on newly emerging diseases. This research has to begin with most fundamental research on the genome of known pathogens and other biological questions that can be studied at the molecular level. If you think that the malaria-carrying Anopheles mosquito, Ebola virus, or Rift Valley fever virus do not seem like important targets for our scientific talent and resources to focus on, you're wrong. There are no longer regional diseases. Every disease can become a global disease. Moreover, the more we learn about current pathogens, the better prepared we'll be for future ones. With a clearer understanding of the real risks involved, the American public would gladly endorse this increase in government spending. Josh Lederberg was right when he first sounded the alarm, and his message has even greater urgency today.

12

Conclusions and Recommendations

I have written this book in the hope of rekindling dialogue on scientific issues related to population. My odyssey through the world of population sciences has led me to key recommendations that I present here in abbreviated form and in greater detail throughout the preceding chapters.

The gap between rich and poor is widening. Economically privileged countries must increase their commitment and accelerate their efforts to achieve greater international equity in education, health, economic opportunity, and other conditions that influence people's lives.

We have a responsibility to elevate the conditions of life for the world's underprivileged people and to preserve the earth for future generations, leaving it in at least as good shape as we found it. For impoverished, powerless people in economically deprived countries, preserving the earth may be the least of their everyday worries. Each morning they begin a struggle for enough food, clean water, and adequate shelter to protect their families. The affluent, influential, and powerful must understand and act upon the long-term implications of human activities and support evidence-driven decisions and policies.

To meet the challenge of increasing the world's food supply, greater crop yields through safe and acceptable scientific advances in soil nutrients and plant breeding, including modern biotechnology, must be included in the global strategy. If alternative approaches to science-based agricultural research and development are formulated, they should be evaluated.

Feeding the world's people and assuring an adequate supply of fresh water cannot be left to chance. There are three billion additional people about to be born. If they do not have access to food and water, they and a multitude of others will suffer malnutrition and hunger, and political upheavals will ensue. Although the limit in crop yield may have been reached using conventional plant breeding, biotechnology and genetic modification of grains and other food crops have the potential to produce varieties of still-higher yield. Some agro-ecologists claim that producing genetically modified foodstuffs will enrich agribusiness industries and impoverish and destroy small farming operations. Environmentalists believe that genetic modification of plants has untested ecological hazards. Other scientists fear the potential damaging side effects from human consumption of transgenic crops.

Worldwide agreement must soon be reached to stem the global emission of carbon dioxide and other greenhouse gases. Projected levels of climate change could destabilize many regions of the world.

We cannot ignore the burden placed on the earth's resources, environment, and ecological balance caused by overconsumption by the wealthy nations and the increasing resource and energy demands of emerging economies. The prospect of climate change caused by elevating levels of greenhouse gases in the atmosphere is of utmost urgency.

Granted that problems of fairness, measurement, and enforcement exist in the present version of the Kyoto Protocol, but this is one bargaining table we cannot walk away from. Inaction could close the window of opportunity for international cooperation.

The success or failure of the multitude of new urban dwellers at finding stable employment and economic security will affect their living conditions and health, and also will have an impact on political stability.

As the twenty-first century begins, half the world's population is living in urban areas, and for the first time in human history, the world has become more urban than rural. People are drawn to cities for jobs as agricultural employment dwindles and many seek opportunities for richer lives than farming can offer. Accommodating the growing numbers in megacities and other urban centers will require visionary policies to assure that the new urbanites' aspirations are not shattered and that they are not trapped in slums without adequate infrastructure and social services.

Clarifying misunderstandings, adopting a common vocabulary, and re-establishing a partnership with strength and mutual respect between advocates of the new paradigm and the old is vitally important.

Sexual equality is a fundamental goal firmly embedded in several UN conference reports. A landmark success was achieved at the Cairo International Conference on Population and Development, where a just balance in gender roles and women's empowerment replaced concern about the consequences of population growth as the defining issues on the international population agenda. This is the new paradigm, perhaps an inevitable outcome of population programs based on demographic arguments, the old paradigm, which world leaders saw as being concerned more with numbers rather than with the needs of people. The Cairo agenda was adopted almost unanimously by 185 nations. In subsequent years, concern about the consequences of population growth has been labeled the "demographic imperative," a description connoting mild criticism to disapproval.

The zealots who would deny women their reproductive freedom should be opposed by a unified coalition of concerned scientists, feminists leaders, policy advocates, and others working together for sexual equality and women's health and empowerment and for clearer understanding of the global consequences of population growth.

Many zealous antagonists to women's progress are also opposed to a rational consideration of population issues. The following statement appeared in a newsletter circulated by a coalition of extremist groups authorized to attend the UN Special General Assembly convened for an assessment of progress five years after the Cairo conference: "There will be no end to this [population-control agenda] until the UN world community comes to realize that contraception, abortion, and all the other methods of the death culture can only result in due course to euthanasia and even in the eventual disappearance of human society" (*Pro-Family News* (1999: 1)).

Contraceptives must be improved to meet the needs of the world's diverse population. Introducing a choice of more effective methods will advance reproductive freedom and reduce the number of abortions performed in the United States and around the world.

Contraceptive use has spread in recent decades. The methods used differ from country to country, but contraception is nearly always the woman's responsibility. In the United States, even though most couples use contraception, about half of the six million pregnancies that occur each year are unintended and unplanned. Among reversible methods, the pill is the most popular in the United States and believed to be the most effective. Yet, under actual conditions of use, it has a failure rate of 3%. Condom use is associated with a 12% rate of unwanted pregnancy, and other methods such as periodic abstinence (rhythm), the diaphragm, and vaginal spermicides have failure rates of around 20%.

About half of all pregnancies resulting from contraceptive failure are voluntarily terminated.

Acts or threats of violence against those performing abortions, conducting contraceptive research, or providing contraceptive services must be investigated and prosecuted by law enforcement agencies with the same diligence as any other act or threat of terrorism.

Virtually every contraceptive product developed in the past 50 years has been challenged under America's legal system, supporting a major industry created from product-liability litigation. Directors of pharmaceutical companies want to avoid expensive legal battles that generate negative publicity and disrupt corporate tranquility. They are concerned about the violent opposition prompted by research into reproductive health products. Unfortunately, they allow these threats to influence their research agenda.

Small start-up companies are more willing to take the perceived risks of developing income-generating contraceptive products. They should be encouraged to collaborate with experienced research programs funded by nonprofit organizations.

Paradoxically, the three-year period from 2000 to 2002 produced a record number of launches of contraceptive products, largely because of the research efforts of publicly supported programs: new contraceptive implants, an intrauterine system that releases a super-progesterone, a skin patch, a vaginal ring contraceptive, emergency contraceptive products, and mifepristone, the effective and safe medical abortifacient. As the programs that produced these products complete their current research projects, the reluctance of major pharmaceutical companies to work in this field will have its effect on the availability of future contraceptive products that resulted from this research.

New contraceptives are being developed that include additional health benefits. They will be part of the twenty-first century's array of new products.

New contraceptives will need to offer broader product profiles. Couples will be looking for noncontraceptive health benefits, particularly for the prevention of sexually transmitted diseases. High priority should be given to developing a vaginal gel that is microbicidal and spermicidal so that women, on their own initiative, can use a contraceptive that will protect them from sexually transmitted disease. Contraceptives can be designed that would also reduce the risk of cancer, heart disease, or osteoporosis. In fact, such contraceptives already exist. Women using oral contraceptives have a lower risk of ovarian, endometrial, and colon cancer, and of benign breast tumors.

New products can be designed that emphasize menstruation suppression. This option will put women in control of the timing of pregnancy and also of the timing of their periods.

With lower fertility, women have moved from the era of incessant reproduction to an era of incessant menstruation. Yet, if they are not attempting to become pregnant, they have no medical or biological need to menstruate. As fertility continues to decline, women around the world will spend more and more of their reproductive years using contraceptives and less time pregnant or lactating. Many will have 35 or 40 years of menstrual cycles without a pregnancy or with only one or two pregnancies and a brief period or two of lactation. For them, the monthly health-related side effects of menstruation are unnecessary. Today's ovulation-suppressing contraceptives can be used to suppress menstruation.

Biomedical scientists must study the diseases that affect most of the world's people living in less developed regions, and respond to the threat of newly emerging diseases. The United States and other industrialized nations must increase the investment in these research efforts as a moral responsibility and for homeland protection against potential bioterrorism.

A number of new diseases can have an impact on world population. Viral diseases that baffle modern medicine are the greatest threat. Disease is no longer geographically confined. Many are airborne, carried by mosquitoes, birds, or aerosols, and by passengers aboard jetliners. All demand the attention of scientists internationally who now devote

90% of their efforts to understanding and controlling diseases that affect 10% of the world's population.

If a country has one dollar to spend on population, family planning, and development, that dollar should be spent on educating young girls.

The educational transition from illiteracy to mass schooling is the precursor of the transition from high to low fertility and of the economic transition to rising income and affluence, and in that process, girls cannot be left behind.

The children listening to their teachers under a banyan tree or in any other classroom are the key to enhancing the status of women and to a better world. Unfortunately, this idea is not yet rooted sufficiently to affect national actions and international assistance policies.

Experts in many scientific disciplines must continue to analyze the consequences of demographic issues. This is the demographic imperative.

Sound policies can be built on accurate information. If we don't adopt policies that protect the earth for future generations, any victory we experience will be a pyrrhic victory and a twenty-first century disaster for progress in women's empowerment to be gained at a time in history when humanity is faced with staggering tragedies resulting from past environmental or food-policy errors. Gender equity for women is a goal for enabling women to fulfill their aspirations, and to improve the quality of life for themselves and their families, not simply to continue the struggle for survival.

No substitute exists for rigorous science and evidence-based conclusions for the formulation of rational policies on population, environmental issues, food security, and the improvement of the human condition.

In this book, I seek to illustrate that population issues influence our lives in many complex ways and that we cannot push science aside in trying to understand and resolve them. These are global problems that require the attention of global science. Junk science, the sound bites of lobbyists, or the polemics of ideologues are no substitutes for the scientific method.

Think about population issues that will affect your lives and those of your children and grandchildren. Give voice to your views. Population is too important to leave to the politicians.

Data Sources

Statistical information used throughout the book been obtained from the tables in the following publications. This is followed by a listing of the articles that served as source material for each chapter.

Demographic and Health Survey Data. Available on DHS website (www. census.gov.pHdata/publications.html), updated 2001.

Family Planning and Population. A compendium of international statistics. The Population Council, New York, 1996.

Global Trends 2015. A dialogue about the future. U.S. National Intelligence Council, Washington, D.C., 2000.

Least Developed Countries 2000 Report. United Nations Conference on Trade and Development (UNCTAD). United Nations, New York, 2000.

Statistical Abstracts of the United States: 2000 (120th edition). U.S. Bureau of the Census, Washington, D.C., 2000.

United Nations Population Division. World population prospects: The 2001 revision, vol. 1, Comprehensive tables. United Nations, New York, 1999.

United Nations Population Fund. The State of world population. United Nations, New York, 2001.

World Development Report 1999/2000. Entering the 21st century. World Bank, Washington, D.C., first printing, August 1999.

World Development Report 2000/2001. Attacking poverty. World Bank, Washington, D.C., first printing, September 2000.

World Population Profile: 1998. Report WP/98. U.S. Bureau of the Census, Washington, D.C., 1998.

World Resources 2000/2001. United Nations Development Programme and others. UN, New York, First Printing September, 2000.

Chapter References

Introduction

The references in this section provide more detailed information on the history of population policy, the origins and development of the family planning movement, and the landmark United Nations International Conference on Population and Development, Cairo, 1984.

Adamson, D. et al. How Americans view world population issues. Rand, Santa Monica, CA, 2000.

Germaine, A. Addressing the demographic imperative through health, empowerment, and rights: implementation in Bangladesh. Health Transition Review 7 (suppl. 4): 10–14 (1997).

Harkavy, O. Curbing population growth: An insider's perspective on the population movement. New York, Plenum Press, 1995.

Jain, A. Do population policies matter? Population Council, New York, 1998.

Menken, J. World population and U.S. policy: The choices ahead. W.W. Norton, New York, 1986.

Population Reference Bureau. Research findings on the Cairo Consensus. Population Reference Bureau, Washington D.C., 1999.

Raina, B.L. A quest for a small family. Commonwealth Publishers, New Delhi, 1991.

Ross, J., and W.P. Mauldin. Berelson on population. Springer-Verlag, New York, 1988.

Sadik, N. Reproductive health and gender equality in the 21st century. International lecture series on population issues. The John D. and Catherine T. MacArthur Foundation, Chicago, IL, 2000.

Sai, F.T. Where is the population movement going? Cairo's legacy. Health Transition Review 7 (Suppl. 4): 1–9 (1997).

Segal, S.J. Acceptance address, The United Nations Population Award, Mexico City, August 13, 1984. The Population Council, New York, 1984.

Segal, S.J. Population politics: Reflections on the International Population Conference held in Mexico City. Wellesley Alumnae Magazine 69(1): 4–9 (1984).

Sen, A. Population policy: Authoritarianism versus cooperation. International Lecture Series on Population. John D. and Catherine T. MacArthur Foundation, Chicago, August 17, 1995.

Sen, G. et al. Population policies reconsidered: Health. empowerment, and rights. Harvard Series on Population and International Health. Harvard University Press, Cambridge, 1994.

United Nations. Key actions for the further implementation of the Programme of Action of the International Conference on Population and Development. United Nations, New York, 1999.

United Nations Population Fund. The state of the world population: 6 billion, a time for choices. United Nations, New York, 1999.

Chapter 1

The Population Division of the United Nations maintains a comprehensive record of national population statistical reports. Population statistics cited in this chapter are taken from UN Population Division World Population Prospects, the 2001 Revision; the World Population Profile: 1998 issued by the U.S. Department of Commerce. Bureau of the Census, and the World Development Report 2000/2001 of the World Bank. References below provide information concerning population density, urbanization, population age structure, unmet needs for family planning, theories on the relationship between population growth and economic development, the science of population forecasting, and the history of world population.

Adamson, D. et al. How Americans view world population issues. Population Matters; 28, 2000.

CIA, National Intelligence Council. Global Trends 2015. Page 39. Government Printing Office, Washington D.C., 2000.

Coale, A.J., and E Hoover, Population growth and economic development in low-income countries. Princeton University Press, Princeton, NJ, 1958.

Cohen, J. How many people can the earth support? New York, W.W. Norton, 1995.

DHS Comparative Studies. Unmet needs, 1990–1994, Demographic and Health Surveys, Comparative Health Surveys No. 16. Demographic and Health Survey. Calverton, MD, June 1995.

Dodoo, F. et al. Slum residence: Adverse health consequences linked in Kenya. Population Briefs 6 (3): 1–8 (2000).

Ehrlich, P. The population bomb. Ballantine, New York, 1968.

Gelbard, A., C. Haub, M. Kent. World population beyond six billion. Population Bulletin 54 (1) (1999).

Gilbert, G. World population: A reference handbook, contemporary world issues. ABC-CLIO, Santa Barbara, CA, 2001.

Hardin, G. The tragedy of the commons. Science 162: 1243–1248 (1968).

Izazola, H., and C. Marquette. Mexico City: Current demographic and environmental trends. In: People and their planet (eds) Baudot B and W. Moomah, St. Martin's Press, New York, 174–186 1999.

Kelley, A.C. Economic consequences of population change in the third world. Journal of Economic Literature 26 (4): 1688 (1988).

Krishna-Hensel, S. Population and urbanization in the 21st century: India's megacities. In: People and their planets (Baudet B. and W. Moomah, eds). St. Martin's Press, New York, 157–173 1999.

Livi-Bacci, M. A concise history of world population, 2nd ed. Blackwell, Maiden, MA, 1997.

Lutz, W. et al. Frontiers of population forecasting. Population and Development Review 24 (suppl.):1–14 (1998).

Meadows, D.H., D.L. Meadows, J. Randers, and W. Behrens III. The limits to growth: A report for the Club of Rome's Project on the Predicament of Mankind, 2nd ed. Universe Books, New York, 1972.

Norgren, Tiana, Abortion before birth control: The politics of reproduction in postwar Japan. Princeton University Press, Princeton, N.J., 2001.

Pope Paul VI. The encyclical *Humanae Vitae*, reaffirming Papal opposition to all forms of birth control except periodic abstinence. Vatican City, 1968.

Population Division. United Nations, population ageing 1999. United Nations, New York, 1999.

Population Reference Bureau. 2000 World population data sheet. Population Reference Bureau, Washington, D.C., 2000.

The Rockefeller Foundation. High stakes: The United States, global population and our common future. The Rockefeller Foundation, New York, 1997.

Simon, J. The ultimate resource. Princeton University Press, Princeton, NJ, 1996.

Speare, A. Optimal city size and population density for the 21st century. In: Elephants in the Volkswagen (L. Grant, ed). W.H. Freeman, New York, 1992.

Chapter 2

In addition to general articles written for readers without a background in medicine or biological sciences, original articles appearing in professional journals are included in the references for this chapter and the subsequent chapters dealing with biomedical subjects. Readers now have access to most of the scientific literature not only from reference books in libraries, but, through the internet, to original publications in professional journals. This database can be accessed at no cost, courtesy of the U.S. National Library of Medicine by entering www.pubmedcentral.nih.gov *through most search engines.*

Blandau, R.L. Follicular growth, ovulation and egg transport. In: The ovary (Mack, II.C., ed). C.C. Thomas, Springfield, IL, 1968.

Franchi, L.L., A.M. Mandl, and S. Zuckerman, The development of the ovary and the process of oogenesis. In: The Ovary (Zuckerman, S., A.M. Mandl, and P. Eckstein, eds). Academic Press, London, 1962.

Lloyd, C.W., and J.H. Leathem. Physiology of the female reproductive tract. In: Human reproduction and sexual behavior (Lloyd, C.W., ed). Lea and Febiger, Philadelphia, PA, 1964. pp. 70–91.

Mead, M., Coming of age in Samoa. Morrow/Avon, New York, 2001.

Nilsson, L. A child is born. Delacourt Press, New York, 1990.

Reproduction: New developments. Science Magazine 266: 5160 (1994).

Segal, S.J. The testis: Physiology. In: Human reproduction and sexual behavior (Lloyd, C.W., ed). Lea and Febiger, Philadelphia, PA, pp. 65–69, 1964.

Segal, S.J. The physiology of human reproduction. Scientific American 231 (3), (1974). pp. 53–62.

Segal, S.J. Sexual differentiation in vertebrates. In: Origin and evolution of sex (Halvorson, H. and A. Monroy, eds). New York, Alan R. Liss, pp. 263–270, 1985.

Segal, S.J., and W.O. Nelson. Initiation and maintenance of testicular function. In: (Lloyd, C.W., ed). Recent progress in the endocrinology of reproduction. Academic Press, New York, pp. 107–122, 1959.

Steinberger, E., and A. Steinberger. Spermatogenic function of the testis. In: Handbook of physiology, vol. V, 287–393 (Greep, R.O., and E.B. Astwood, eds). Williams and Wilkins, Baltimore, 1975.

Velduls, J. Pituitary-testicular axis. In: Reproductive endocrinology (Yen, S.S., and R.B. Jaffe, eds). W.B. Saunders, Philadelphia, PA, 1991.

Woodburne, R.T. Essentials of human anatomy. Oxford University Press, New York, 1965.

Yen, S.S., and R.B. Jaffe. Reproductive endocrinology. W.B. Saunders Company, Philadelphia, 1978.

Chapter 3

These references contain information about the evolutionary history of the human reproductive system, the impact of menstruation on women's health including ovarian cancer and endometriosis, theories pertaining to the nonreproductive role of menstruation, and methods women can use to control their own menstruation. Women's attitudes toward menstruation are also recorded.

Andersson, K., and G. Rybo. Levonorgestrel-releasing intrauterine device in the treatment of mennorhagia. British Journal of Obstetrics and Gynaecology 97: 690–694 (1990).

Arumugam, K., and J. Lim. Menstrual characteristics associated with endometriosis. British Journal of Obstetrics and Gynaecology 104 (8): 948–950 (1997).

Bruner, A. et al. Randomized study of cognitive effects of iron supplementation in non-anemic, iron deficient girls. The Lancet 348: 992–996 (1996).

Casagrande, J. Incessant ovulation and ovarian cancer. The Lancet 316: 170–173 (1979).

Case, A., and R. Reid. Effects of the menstrual cycle on medical disorders. Archives of Internal Medicine 158: 1405–1412 (1998).

Centers for Disease Control and NICHD. The reduction of risk of ovarian cancer associated with oral contraceptive use. New England Journal of Medicine 316: 650–655 (1987).

Contraceptive Technology Update. Research eyes extending the menstrual cycle. Monthly Newsletter of American Health Consultants, Atlanta, GA, vol. 23, no. 1, 2002.

Coutinho, E., and S.J. Segal. Is menstruation obsolete? Oxford University Press, New York, 1999.

Darrow, S., J. Vena, E. Batt, et al. Menstrual characteristics and the risk of endometriosis. Epidemiology 4 (2): 135–142 (1993).

Den Tonkelaar, L., and B. Oddens. Preferred frequency and characteristics on menstrual bleeding in relation to reproductive status, oral contraceptive use, and hormone replacement therapy use. Contraception 59: 357–362 (1999).

Houppert, K. The curse: Confronting the last unmentionable taboo, menstruation. Farrar, Straus & Giroux, New York, 1999.

Howell, N. Demography of the Dobe! Kung. University of Toronto Press, Toronto, 1979.

Kristjansdottir, J., E. Johansson, and L. Ruusavaara. The cost of the menstrual cycle in young Swedish women. European Journal of Contraception and Reproductive Health Care 5: 152–156 (2000).

Lahteenmaki, P., M. Haukkamaa, J. Poulakka, et al. Open randomized study of use of levonorgestrel releasing intrauterine system as alternative to hysterectomy. British Medical Journal 316: 112–126 (1998).

La Vecchia, C., S. Franceschi, G. Gallus, et al. Incessant ovulation and ovarian cancer: a critical approach. International Journal of Epidemiology 12 (2): 161–164 (1983).

Miller, L., and K. Notter. Menstrual reduction with extended use of combined oral contraceptive pills: Randomized controlled trial. Obstetrics and Gynecology 98: 771–778 (2001).

Profit, M. Menstruation as a defense against pathogens transported by sperm. The Quarterly Review of Biology 68 (3): 335–381 (1993).

Short, R. Human reproduction in an evolutionary context. Annals of the New York Academy of Sciences 709: 416–425 (1994).

Snowden R., and B. Christian, eds. Patterns and perceptions of menstruation. A World Health Organization international study. St. Martin's Press, New York, 1983.

Sobo, E. Menstruation: an ethno-physiological defense against pathogens. Perspectives in Biology and Medicine 8: 36–39 (1994).

Strassmann, B. The evolution of endometrial cycles and menstruation. The Quarterly Review of Biology 71: 181–220 (1996).

Strassmann, B. Menstrual cycling and breast cancer: an evolutionary perspective. Journal of Women's Health 8 (2): 193–202 (1999).

Thomas, S., and C. Ellertson. Nuisance or natural and healthy: Should monthly menstruation be optional for women? Lancet 355: 922–924 (2000).

Treloar, A., R. Boynton, B. Benn, and B. Brown, Variation in human menstrual cycle throughout reproductive life. International Journal of Fertility 12: 77 (1967).

Vercellini, P., O. DeGiorgi, G. Aimi, et al. Menstrual characteristics in women with and without endometriosis. Obstetrics and Gynecology 90 (2): 264–268 (1997).

Chapter 4

These references document information on the history of contraception prior to the 1960, the development of the pill, and the controversy surrounding this historical breakthrough. References are included on modern thinking regarding the risks and benefits of oral contraceptive use. The citations also provide more detailed information on the emergence of modern intrauterine devices.

Asbell, B. The pill: A biography of the drug that changed the world. Random House, New York, 1995.

Beral, V., C. Hermon, C. Kay, et al. Mortality associated with oral contraceptive use: 25 years follow up of cohort of 46,000 women from Royal College of General Practitioners' oral contraceptive study. British Medical Journal 318: 96–1000 (1999).

Dizfalusy, E. The contraception revolution: An era of scientific and social achievement. CRC Press, Boca Raton, FL, 1997.

Djerassi, C. The politics of contraception. W.W. Norton & Company, New York, 1980.

Edwards, R., and J. Cohen. Reproductive choices in 2000: The relative safety of current oral contraceptives. Human Reproduction Update 5 (6): 563–564 (2000).

Grimes, D. Long-term reversible contraception. Twelve years of experience with the TCu380A and TCu220C. Contraception 56: 341–352 (1997).

Himes, N. Medical history of contraception. Gamut Press, New York, 1936/1963.

Kemmeren, J., A. Algra, and D. Grobbee. Third generation oral contraceptives and the risk of venous thrombosis: Meta-analysis, British Medical Journal 323 (7305): 131–134 (2001).

Lee, N.C., G. Rubin, and R. Borucki. The intrauterine device and pelvic inflammatory disease revisited: New results from the Women's Health Study. Obstetrics and Gynecology 72: 1–6 (1988).

Mauldin, W.P., and S.J. Segal. Prevalence of contraceptive use: Trends and issues. Studies in Family Planning 19: 335–353 (1988).

McLaughlin, L. The pill, John Rock, and the church, Little, Brown and Company, Boston, MA, 1982.

Population Council. The Copper T380 intrauterine device: A summary of scientific data. Population Council, New York, 1994.

Poulter, N., C. Chang, M. Marmot, T. Farley, and O. Meirik. Third generation oral contraceptives and venous thrombosis. 349 (9053): 732 (1997).

Rock, J. The time has come. Avon Books, New York, 1964.

Segal, S.J. Trends in population and contraception. Journal of Reproductive Medicine 1 (2): 93–106 (1992).

Segal, S.J. Gregory Pincus, father of the pill. Population Today, Population Reference Bureau, Washington, D.C., vol. 28: no. 5, July 2000.

Segal, S.J., F. Alvarez, and C. Adejuwon. Absence of chorionic gonadotrophin in sera of women who use intrauterine devices. Fertility and Sterility 44 (2): 214–218 (1985).

Snow, Edgar. The other side of the river. Random House, New York, 1967.

Spitzer, W. Balanced view of risks of oral contraceptives. Lancet 350 (9091): 1566–1567 (1997).

Vessey, M. Oral contraception and health. British Journal of General Practice 48 (435): 1639–40 (1998).

Weiss, G. Risk of venous thromboembolism with third generation oral contraceptives: a review. American Journal of Obstetrics and Gynecology, 180 (2): 295–301 (1999).

World Health Organization. Mechanism of action, safety and efficacy of intrauterine devices. Technical Report Series 753. World Health Organization, Geneva, 1987.

World Health Organization Scientific Group. Cardiovascular disease and steroid hormone contraception. WHO Technical Report Series, 877. World Health Organization, Geneva, 1998.

Chapter 5

The arguments for the need for new and improved contraceptives are contained in the following references. Citations provide considerable detail on Norplant implants and IUD improvements. Current concepts on the safety of IUDs are described. The citations also include information on the new contraceptive methods introduced in the United States 2000–2002 as well as methods still under investigation.

Al Azhar University. Personal visit by S.J. Segal: approval for study of Norplant. (Al Azhar is one of the oldest Islamic academic institutions. It acts as an authority on Qu'ranic interpretation and policy making.) Al Azhar University, Cairo, 1986.

Apter, D., et al. Clinical performance and endocrine profiles of contraceptive vaginal ring releasing 3-keto-desogestrel and ethinyl estradiol. Contraception. 42 (3): 285–295 (1990).

Baulieu, E.E., and S.J. Segal, eds. The antiprogestin steroid RU 486 and human fertility control. Plenum Press, New York, 1985.

Berlex Laboratories, Inc. Fact Sheet: Mirena®: Two decades in development, ten years practical experience. Berlex Laboratories, Montville, NJ, 2000.

Bongaarts, J., and E. Johansson. Future trends in contraception and reproductive health products. Population Briefs, vol. 2 (4). Population Council, New York, 1996.

Bygdeman, M., and M. Swahn. Progesterone receptor blockage—effect on uterine contractility and early pregnancy. Contraception 32: 45–51 (1985).

Contraceptive Technology Update. First contraceptive patch offers once-a-week dosing. Monthly Newsletter of American Health Consultants, Atlanta, GA, vol. 23, no.1, 2002.

Coutinho, E., et al. A comparative study of intermittent vs. continuous use of a contraceptive pill administered by vaginal route. Contraception 51: 355 (1995).

Creasy, G., N. Hall, and G. Shangold. Patient adherence with the contraceptive patch dosing schedule vs. oral contraceptives. Obstetrics and Gynecology 95 (4, suppl. 1): S60 (2000).

Davies, G., et al. Ovarian activity and bleeding patterns during extended continuous use of a combined contraceptive vaginal ring. Contraception 46 (3): 269–278 (1992).

Fotherby, K., et al. A pharmacological trial of the monthly injectable contraceptive cycloprovera. Contraception 25 (3): 261–272 (1982).

Hatcher, R. Depo-Provera®. Norplant®, and progestin only pills (minipills). In: Contraceptive technology, 17th ed. (Hatcher, R., et al., eds). 1998; pp. 467–509.

Kaunitz, A. Injectable Depot Medroxyprogesterone Acetate Contraception: An update for U.S. Clinicians. International Journal of Fertility 43 (2): 73–83 (1998).

Kiriwat, A., and H. Coelingh-Bennick. A 4-year pilot study on the efficacy and safety of Implanon®. European Journal of Contraception and Reproductive Health Care 3: 85–91 (1998).

Lahteenmaki, P., M. Kaukkamaa, J. Puolakka, U. Riikonen, S. Sainio, J. Overbaugh, and D. Panteleeff. Open randomized study of the use of levonorgestrel releasing intrauterine system as alternative to hysterectomy. British Medical Journal 316: 1122–1126 (1998).

Newhall, E., and B. Winikoff. Abortion with mifepristone and misoprostol: Regimens, efficacy, acceptability and future directions. American Journal of Obstetrics and Gynecology 183 (2, suppl.): S44–S53 (2000).

Naz, R.K. Vaccine for contraception targeting sperm. Immunological Reviews 171: 193–202 (1999).

Oliveras E., et al. Jadelle® two-rod contraceptive implants. Johns Hopkins Program for International Education in Gynecology and Obstetrics, Baltimore, MD, 1998.

Organon Inc. Fact Sheet; Nuvaring®: The first monthly vaginal ring for birth control receives FDA approval. Organon Inc, West Orange, NJ, 2001.

Ortho-McNeil Pharmaceuticals. Ortho Evra™ the first birth control patch. Ortho-McNeil Pharmaceuticals, Raritan, NJ, 2001.

Polaneczky, M., et al. The use of levonorgestrel implants (Norplant®) for contraception in adolescent mothers. New England Journal of Medicine 331: 1201–1206 (1994).

Population Council. The levonorgestrel releasing intrauterine system: A contraceptive and reproductive health product. Population Briefs, vol. 2, no. 4. Population Council, New York, 1996.

Pymar, H., and M. Creinin. Alternatives to mifepristone regimens for medical abortion. American Journal of Obstetrics and Gynecology 183 (2, suppl.): S54–S65 (2000).

Roddy, R.E., L. Zekeng, K. Ryan, U. Tamoufé, and K. Tweedy. Effect of nonoxynol-9 on genital gonorrhea and chlamydial infection. Journal of the American Medical Association 287 (9): 1117–1122 (2002).

Schindler, A. The 3-keto-desorgestrel/ethinyl-estradiol ring: a new parenteral form of hormonal contraception. European Journal of Obstetrics and Gynecology Reproductive Biology 49 (1–2): 13–14 (1993).

Segal, S.J. What's the latest on IUDs? Contemporary Obstetrics and Gynecology 16:115–118 (1980).

Segal, S.J. The development of NORPLANT® Implants. Studies in Family Planning 14 (6/7): 159–163 (1983).

Segal, S.J. Seeking better contraceptives. Populi 11 (2): 24–30 (1984).

Segal, S.J. A new delivery system for contraceptive steroids. American Journal of Obstetrics and Gynecology 157: 1090–1097 (1987).

Segal, S.J. Contraceptive innovations: needs and opportunities. In: Demographic and Programmatic Consequences of Contraceptive Innovations (Segal, S.J., A. Tsui, and S. Rogers, eds). Plenum Press, New York, pp. 3–32 1989.

Segal, S.J., et al. Norplant implants: The mechanism of contraceptive action. Fertility and Sterility 56(2): 272–277 (1991).

Segal, S.J. The future of contraception. In: Reproductive medicine and surgery (Wallach, E., and H. Zacur, eds). Mosby, Baltimore, MD, pp. 351–362, 1994.

Segal, S.J. Contraceptive development and better family planning. Bulletin of the New York Academy of Medicine 73(1): 92–104 (1996).

Spitz, I., C.W. Bardin, L. Benton, and A. Robbins. Early pregnancy termination with mifepristone and misoprostol in the United States. New England Journal of Medicine 338: 1241–1247 (1998).

Stevens, V.C. Progress in the development of human chorionic gonadotropin antifertility vaccines. American Journal of Reproductive Immunology 35: 148–155 (1996).

Talwar, G.P. A vaccine that prevents pregnancy in women. Proceedings of the National Academy of Sciences, USA vol. 94: 8532–8536 (1994).

Talwar, G.P. Vaccines and passive immunological approaches for the control of fertility and hormone-dependent cancers. Immunological Reviews 171: 173–192 (1999).

Van de Wijgert,-J. and C. Coggins. Microbicides to prevent heterosexual transmission of HIV: Ten years down the road. AIDS science (1): 2002. Available at www.aidscience.com.

Chapter 6

References discuss the general issue of developing contraceptives for use by men; the use of gossypol as a male contraceptive; oral or systemic use of androgens and progestins to suppress spermatogenesis; and studies with 7 α-methyl-19 nor testosterone.

Alvarez-Sanchez, F., Faundes, V. Brache, and P. Leon, Attainment and maintenance of azoospermia with combined monthly infections of depot-medroxyprogesterone acetate and testosterone enanthate. Contraception 15: 635–647 (1977).

Bain, J, V. Rachlis, K. Roberts, and Z. Khait, The combined use of oral medroxyprogesterone acetate and methyl testosterone in a male contraceptive trial program. Contraception 21: 356–379 (1980).

Bardin, C.W., R. Swerdloff, and R. Santen. Androgens: Risks and benefits. Journal of Clinical Endocrinology and Metabolism. 73 (4): 4–7 (1991).

Coutinho, E, F. Alvarez, M. Reidenberg, and S.J. Segal. Gossypol levels and inhibition of spermatogenesis in men taking gossypol as a contraceptive. Contraception 61: 61–67 (2000).

Coutinho, E.M., and J.F. Melo. Successful inhibition of spermatogenesis in men without loss of libido: A potential new approach to male contraception. Contraception 8: 207–217 (1973).

Family Health International. Men and reproductive health. Family Health International, Research Triangle Park, NC, 1998.

Foegh, M. Evaluation of steroids as contraceptives in man. Acta Endocrinologica 104 (suppl. 260): 1–48 (1983).

Frick, J. Control of spermatogenesis in men by combined administration of progestin and androgen. Contraception 8: 191–206 (1973).

Gu, Z.P., Segal, S.J., and M.M. Reidenberg. Serum potassium: Values in normal men in Shanghai vs. men from Shanghai living abroad. Clinical Chemistry 40: 350 (1994).

Guerin, J.F., and J. Rollet. Inhibition of spermatogenesis in men using various combinations of oral progestogens and percutaneous or oral androgens. International Journal of Andrology 11: 187–199 (1988).

Handelsman, D., A. Conway, L. Boylan. Suppression of human spermatogenesis by testosterone implants. Journal of Clinical Endocrinology and Metabolism 75: 1326–32 (1992).

Hershlag A, Cooper G, and S. Benoff. Pregnancy following discontinuation of a calcium channel blocker in a the male partner. Human Reproduction; 10(3): 599–606 (1995).

Koide, S.S., et al. Antisperm antibodies associated with infertility: Properties and encoding genes of target antigens. Proceeding of the Society of Experimental Biology 22: 1–47 (2000).

Kumar N., A. Didolkar, C. Monder, C.W. Bardin, and K. Sundaram. The biological activity of 7α-methyl-19-nortestosterone is not amplified in the male reproductive tract as is that of testosterone. Endocrinology 130: 3677–3683 (1992).

National Coordinating Group on Male Infertility Agents. A new anti-fertility agent for males. Chinese Medical Journal 4: 417 (1978).

Nieschlag, E., H. Hoogen, H. Bolk, H. Schuster, and E. Wickings. Clinical trials with testosterone undecanoate for male fertility control. Contraception 18: 607–614 (1978).

Noé G, J. Suvisaari, C. Martin, A. Moo-Young, K. Sundaram, S. Saleh, E. Quintero, H. Croxatto, and P. Lahteenmaki. Gonadotrophin and testosterone suppression by 7α-methyl-19-nortestosterone acetate administered by subdermal implant to healthy men. Human Reproduction 14: 2200–2206 (1999).

Polsky, B. S.J. Segal, P. Baron, J. Gold, H. Ueno, and D. Armstrong. Inactivation of human immunodeficiency virus in vitro by gossypol. Contraception 29: 18–23 (1989).

Qian, S.Z., and Z.G. Wang, Gossypol: A potential antifertility agent for males. Annual Review of Pharmacology and Toxicity 24: 329–360 (1984).

Reddy, P.R.K., and J.M. Rao, Reversible antifertility action of testosterone propionate in human males. Contraception 5: 295–301 (1972).

Segal, S.J. Contraceptive research: A male chauvinist plot? Family Planning Perspectives 4(3): 21–25 (1972).

Segal, S.J., ed. Gossypol: A potential contraceptive for men. Plenum Press, New York, 1986.

Sundaram, K., et al. 7α methyl-19-nortestosterone (MENT®): The optimal androgen for male contraception. Annals of Medicine 25: 199–205 (1993).

Suvisaaari, J., K. Sundaram, G. Noé, N. Kumar, C. Aguillaume, Y.Y. Tsong, P. Latheenmaki, and C.W. Bardin. Pharmacokinetics and pharmacodynamics of 7α-methyl-19-nortestosterone (MENT) after intramuscular administration in healthy men. Human Reproduction 12: 967–973 (1997).

Wang, C., and K. Yeung. Use of low dosage oral cyproterone acetate as a male contraceptive. Contraception 21: 245–72 (1980).

World Health Organization Task Force on Methods for the Regulation of Male Fertility. Contraceptive efficacy of testosterone-induced azoospermia in normal men. Lancet 336: 955–959 (1990).

World Health Organization Task Force on Methods for the Regulation of Male Fertility. Rates of testosterone induced severe oligospermia in two multinational clinical studies. International Journal of Andrology 18: 1577–1565 (1995).

Chapter 7

These citations provide detailed information on the scientific, legal, and corporate constraints that impede contraceptive research. Comparison in attitudes toward contraceptive research between the pharmaceutical companies of the United States and those of Europe and elsewhere can be found, along with an explanation for the differences.

Institute of Medicine. Contraceptive research and development: Looking to the future (P. Harrison and A.G. Rosenfield, eds). National Academy of Sciences Press, Washington, D.C., 1998.

Institute of Medicine. Contraceptive research, introduction and use: Lessons from Norplant. National Academy Press, Washington, D.C., 1998.

Kolata, G. Will the lawyers kill off Norplant? New York Times, p. 11, May 3, 1995.

The Rockefeller Foundation. Proceedings of the Bellagio Conference on Comparative Aspects of Contraceptive Availability. The Rockefeller Foundation, New York, October 14–18, 1996.

Segal, S.J. The development of modern contraceptive technology. Technology in Society 9: 277–282 (1987).

Segal, S.J. The role of technology in population policy. Populi, vol. 18, no. 4, pp. 5–13, United Nations, New York, 1991.

Segal, S.J. Contraceptive update. Review of Law and Social Change 23(3): 457–469 1998.

Chapter 8

These citations trace the attitudes and predications about the adequacy of food production and the problem of unequal distribution. The ci-

tations include references to both sides of the debate about applying modern biotechnology to food products to meet increased demands and emphasizes work published on golden rice to illustrate this issue. References are also included that describe in greater detail the shortage of fresh water that looms ahead.

Altieri, M. Applying agroecology to enhance the productivity of peasant farming systems in Latin America. Environment, Development, and Sustainability 1: 191–217 (1999).

Barrion, A.T., and J.A. Litsinger. Riceland spiders of South and Southeast Asia. CAB International, Wallingford, U.K., 1995.

Borlaug, N.E. Ending world hunger: the promise of biotechnology and the threat of antiscience zealotry. Plant Physiology 124: 487–490 (2000).

Boserup, E. 1963 Essay on the conditions of agricultural growth: The economics of agrarian change under population pressure. Earthscan Publications, London, 1993.

Burkhardt, P., P. Beyer, J. Wünn, A. Klöti, G. Armstrong, M Schledt, J. von Lintig, I. Potrykus. Transgenic rice (Oryza sativa) endosperm expressing daffodil (Narcissus pseudonarcissus) phytoene synthase accumulates phytoene, a key intermediate of provitamin A biosynthesis. Plant Journal 11: 1071–1078 (1997).

Chrispeels, M.J. Biotechnology and the poor. Plant Physiology 124: 3–6 (2000).

Chistensen, J. Golden rice in a grenade-proof greenhouse. New York Times, p. 36, November 21, 2000.

Coghlan, S. Filling the bowl: For billions worldwide, a modified grain could end lean times. New Scientist Vol. 166 (2232); 19 April 1 (2000).

Conway, G. The doubly green revolution: Food for all in the 21st century. Penguin Books, London, 1997.

Conway, G. Letter to D. Parr, Greenpeace, January 22, 2001. Rockefeller Foundation, New York, 2001.

Conway, G., and G. Toenniessen. Feeding the world in the twenty-first century. Nature 402 (7661 suppl): C55–58 (1999).

Cook, R.J. Science-based risk assessment for the approval and use of plants in agriculture and other environments. In: Agricultural biotechnology and the poor: proceedings of an international conference (Persley, G.J., and M.M. Lantin, eds). Consultative Group on International Agricultural Research, Washington, D.C., pp 16–31 2000.

Dyson, T. Population and food. Routledge Press, London, 1996.

Ellstrand, N., H. Prentice, and J. Hancock. Gene flow and introgression from domesticated plants into their wild relatives. Annual Review of Ecology and Systematics 30: 539–63 (1999).

Evans, L.T. Feeding the ten billion: Plants and population growth. Cambridge University Press, Cambridge.

Gleick, P. The human right to water. Water Policy 1(5) (1999).

Gleick, P. The changing water paradigm: A look at twenty-first century water resources development. Water International 25: 1 (2000).

Goto, F., T. Yoshihara, N. Shigemoto, S. Toki, and F. Takaiwa. Iron fortification of rice seed by the soybean ferritin gene. Nature Biotechnology 17(3): 282–286.

Greenpeace. Genetically engineered "golden rice" is fool's gold. Greenpeace, Manila/Amsterdam, February 9, 2001.

Guerinot, M.L. The green revolution strikes gold. Science 287: 241–243 (2000).

Johnson, S. The green revolution. Harper Torch Books, New York, 1972.

Ku, M., M. Miyano, and M. Matsuoka. Insertion of maize C-4 genes into C-3 rice plants. Nature Biotechnology 17: 76 (2000).

Malthus, T.R. 1798. Essay on the principle of population chapter 2. In: Oxford's world's classics (G. Geoffrey, ed). Oxford University Press, 1998.

May, R. Genetically modified foods: facts, worries, policies and public confidence. Office of Science and Technology, London, 1999.

Mikkelson, T., B. Anderson, and R. Jorgenson. The risk of crop transgene spread. Nature 380 (6569): 31 (1996).

Nash, J.M. Grains of hope. Time Magazine, July 31, 2000, pp. 38–46.

Nuffield Council on Bioethics. Genetically modified crops: the ethical and social issues. Nuffield Council on Bioethics, London; 1999.

Paarlberg, R. The global food fight. In: Foreign affairs, vol. 79, no. 3. Council on Foreign Relations, New York, May/June 2000.

Paddock, W., and P. Paddock, Famine, 1975! America's decision: Who will survive? Little, Brown, Boston, MA, 1967.

Pinstrup-Anderson, P., R. Pandya-Lorch, and M.W. Rosegrant. World food prospects: critical issues of the early twenty-first century. International Food Policy Research Institute, Washington, D.C., 1999.

Population Reference Bureau. South Africa's water policy champions rights of people and ecosystems. Population Today, vol. 28, no. 5. Population Reference Bureau, Washington, D.C., 2000.

Postel, S. Water, Food, and Population. In: People and their planet (B. Baudot and W. Moomah, eds). St. Martin's Press, New York, 1999.

Postel, S.L., C. Gretchen, and P. Ehrlich. Human appropriation of renewable fresh water. Science 271: 785–788 (1996).

Potrykus, I. Golden rice and beyond. Plant Physiology, 125: 1157–1161 (2001).

Sahai, S. Bt Cotton: Confusion prevails. Economic and Political Weekly, May 25, 2002.

Somerville, C. The genetically modified organism conflict. Plant Physiology 123: 1201–1202 (2000).

Tropical Soil Biology and Fertility Programme. Integrating soils, systems and society: TSBF's contribution to integrated, natural resource management research 2001–2005. Tropical Soil Biology and Fertility Programme, Nairobi, 2002.

United Nations Food and Agriculture Organization. The Rome Declaration on World Food Security. Food and Agriculture Organization, Rome, 1996.

Victor, D and C. Runge. Sustaining a revolution: a policy strategy for crop engineering. A Council on Foreign Relations Paper, New York, NY, 2002.

Working Group of the Royal Society of London, the U.S. National Academy of Sciences, the Brazilian Academy of Sciences, the Chinese Academy of Sciences, the Indian National Science Academy, the Mexican Academy of Sciences and the Third World Academy of Sciences. Transgenic plants and world agriculture. National Academy Press, Washington, D.C., 2000.

Ye, X., S. Al-Babili, A. Kloti, J. Zhang, P. Lucca, P. Beyer, and I. Potrykus. Engineering the provitamin A (beta-carotene) biosynthesis pathway into (carotenoid-free) rice endosperm. Science 287 (5451): 303–305 (2000).

Chapter 9

Two topics are emphasized in these references: greenhouse gas emissions (climate change), and pollution of the world's waters. Data concerning atmospheric pollution are taken primarily from the report of the Intergovernmental Panel on Climate Change.

Ayres, R.U. How economists have misjudged global warming. World Watch September/October 2001.

Carson, Rachel. Silent spring. Houghton Mifflin, Boston, MA, 1962.

Cifuentes, L., et al. Hidden health benefits of greenhouse gas mitigation. Science v. 293 (5533) 1257–1259 (2001).

DeLeo, G.A., et al. The economic benefits of the Kyoto Protocol. Nature 4: 478–479 (2001).

de Serbinin, A. Two threats to global security. In: People and their planet (B. Baudot and W. Moomah, eds). St. Martin's Press, New York, 1999.

Dickey, C., and A. Rogers. Smoke and mirrors. Newsweek, February 25, 2002, pp. 30–32.

Environmental Protection Agency. United States Climate Action Report 2002. U.S. Government Printing Office, Washington, D.C., June, 2002.

Gleick, P. The world's water 2000–2001. Island Press, Washington, D.C., 2000.

Helvarg, D. Blue frontier: Saving America's living seas. W.H. Freeman, New York, 2001.

Intergovernmental Panel on Climate Change. Climate change 2001: Impacts, adaptation, and vulnerability. IPCC, Geneva, 2001.

International Herald Tribune. European Union agrees to sign Kyoto climate pact. Paris, March 5, 2002.

Jordan, N.J. Population, environment and sustainable development: Global issues. In: People and their planet (B. Baudot and W. Moomah, eds). St. Martin's Press, New York, 1999.

Marland, G., T.A. Boden, R.C. Griffin, et al. Estimates pf CO2 emissions from fossil fuel burning. Oak Ridge National Laboratory, Oak Ridge, Tennessee, 1993.

CIA, National Intelligence Council. Global Trends 2015. Government Printing Office, Washington, D.C., 2000.

McNeil, J.R. Something new under the sun: An environmental history of the twentieth century. W.W. Norton, New York, 2001.

Moomah, W., and D. Tullis. Population, affluence or technology? An empirical look at national carbon dioxide production. In: People and their planet (B. Baudot and W. Moomah, eds). St. Martin's Press, New York, 1999.

NRC, Committee on the Science of Climate Change. Climate change science: An analysis of some key questions. National Research Council, Washington, D.C., 2001.

Ness, G.D., W.D. Drake, and S.R. Brechin, eds. Population-environment dynamics: Ideas and observations. University of Michigan Press, Ann Arbor, 1993.

O'Neill, B., et al. Population and climate change. Cambridge University Press, Cambridge, 2001.

Popely, R. Carmakers move toward hydrogen fuel cells. Chicago Tribune, August 12, 2001.

Revkin, A. 178 nations reach a climate accord; U.S. only looks on. New York Times, July 24, 2001.

Revkin, A. Climate changing, U.S. Says in Report. New York Times. p. 1, June 3, 2002.

White, R.M. The great climate debate. Scientific American July (1990).

World Commission on Dams. Dams and development; a new framework for decision-making. Earthscan, London, 2000.

World Resources Institute. Carbon counts: Estimating climate change mitigation in foresting projects. World Resources Institute, New York, 1997.

Chapter 10

Key references are provided concerning the importance of education for reducing fertility. Special attention is given to source material on violence against women, including female genital mutilation. Legal efforts to promote reproductive rights are also covered.

Amnesty International. Female genital mutilation: A human rights information pack. Amnesty International, London, 1997.

Askin, K. Sexual violence in decisions and indictments of the Yugoslav and Rwandan tribunals: current status. American Journal of International Law 93: 97–98 (1991).

Center for Reproductive Law and Policy. Promoting reproductive rights: A global mandate. CRLP, New York, 1997.

Center for Reproductive Law and Policy. Reproductive rights 2000: Moving forward. CRLP, New York, 2000.

Jejeebhoy, S. Women's education, autonomy, and reproductive behaviour. Clarendon Press, Oxford, 1995.

Knodel, J. and G. Jones. Does promoting girl's schooling miss the mark? Population and Development Review 4: 683–702 (1996).

Lloyd, C. The spread of primary schooling in sub-Saharan Africa: Implications for fertility change. Population and Development Review 26 (3): 483–515 (2000).

Rahman, A., and N. Toubia. Female genital mutilation: a guide to laws and policies worldwide. Zed Books, New York, 2000.

Sadik, N. Reproductive health and gender equality in the 21st century. International Lecture Series on Population, The John D. and Catherine T. Mac Arthur Foundation, New York, July 3, 2000.

Shalov, C. Rights to sexual and reproductive health: The ICPD and the elimination of all forms of discrimination against women. Health and Human Rights 4(2): 117–127 2000.

Toubia, N., and S. Izett. Female genital mutilation: an overview. World Health Organization, Geneva, 1998.

United Nations General Assembly. Traditional or customary practices affecting the health of women. Report of the Secretary General, 53rd session, September 10, 1998.

Chapter 11

References on HIV/AIDS are emphasized in the following list. There are also key references to major killer diseases that are linked to environmental hazards but do not receive as much public attention and to the threat of newly emerging infection diseases.

Ames, B.N. Identifying environmental chemicals causing mutations and cancer. Science 11: 587–593 (1979).

Chen, L., J. Sepulveda, and S. Segal. AIDS and women's reproductive health. Plenum Press, New York, 1991.

Coggins, C., and S. Segal. AIDS and reproductive health. Journal of Immunology 41: 3–15 (1998).

Dye, C. et al. Global burden of tuberculosis: Estimated incidence, prevalence, and mortality by country. Journal of American Medical Association 282: 677–686 (1999).

Garrett, L. The coming plague: Newly emerging diseases in a world out of order. Penguin Books, New York, 1995.

Hughes, W.W. Essentials of environmental toxicity: their effects of environmentally hazardous substances on human health. Taylor & Francis, Washington, D.C., 1996.

Marmot, M., and R. Wilkinson. Social determinants of health. Oxford University Press, Oxford, 1999.

McNeil, W.H. Plagues and people. Anchor Press/Doubleday, Garden City, New York, 1976.

Morse, S.S., ed. Emerging viruses. Oxford University Press, New York, 1993.

Oldstone, M. Viruses, plagues, and history. Oxford University Press, New York, 1998.

Pope, C. A., R. Burnett, M. Thun, E. Calle, D. Krewski, K. Ito, and G. Thurston. Lung cancer, cardiopulmonary mortality, and long-term exposure to fine particle air pollution. Journal of the American Medical Association 287 (9): 1132–1141 (2002).

Prusiner, S. Molecular biology of prion diseases. Science Magazine 252: 1515–1522 (1991).

Prusiner, S. The prion diseases. Scientific American 272(1): 48–57 (1995).

Rose, J., ed. Environmental toxicology: current developments. Gordon and Breach, London, U.K., 1998.

Stanecki, E.A., and P. Way. The demographic impacts of HIV/AIDS. Perspectives from World Population Profile: 1996. IPC Staff Paper no. 86. U.S. Bureau of the Census, Washington, D.C., 1997.

U.N. AIDS, Table of country-specific HIV/AIDS estimates and data. United Nations Programme on AIDS, Geneva, 2001.

United Nations Environment Programme. Rio declaration of environment and development. United Nations, New York, 2001.

World Health Organization, Tuberculosis—Fact sheet no. 104, revised April 2000. World Health Organization, Geneva, 2000.

World Health Organization. Global tuberculosis control, WHO, Geneva, 2001.

World Health Organization. HIV, TB, and malaria: Diseases of poverty that block social and economic growth. WHO, Geneva, 2001.

Chapter 12

Although this section of the book draws from information given in previous chapters, additional references are included because they have provided insights that are pervasive throughout the book. For readers interested in a more detailed discussion of globalization by its proponents and opponents, these references will be useful.

Bello, W. The future in the balance: Essays on globalization and resistance. Food First Books, Oakland, CA, 2001.

Berelson, B., R. Anderson, and O. Harkavy. Family planning and population programs: A review of world developments. University of Chicago Press, Chicago, 1965.

Bongaarts, J. The role of family planning programmes in contemporary fertility transitions. In: The continuing demographic transition (Jones, G., et al. eds). Oxford University Press, New York, 1997.

Caldwell, J.C. Theory of fertility decline. Academic Press, New York, 1982.

Friedman, T. The Lexus and the olive tree. Anchor Books, New York, 2000.

Livi Bacci, M., and G. DeSantis, eds. Population and poverty in the developing world. Clarendon Press, Oxford, 1999.

Nye, J.S. Jr. Globalization's democratic deficit. Foreign Affairs 80(4): 2–7 (2001).

Pro-Family News. "Vivant!" Special edition, vol. 1, no. 6, March 30, 1999.

Scott, B.R. The great divide in the global village. Foreign Affairs 80(1): 160–177 (2001).

Sen, A. Population: Delusion and reality. New York Review of Books, September 22, 1994, pp. 62–70.

Sen, A. Development as freedom. Alfred Knopf, New York, 1999.

Index

233

238   *Index*

population growth, 199
water problems, 159–160
Mexico City Conference 1984, xxii
Micro-loans, xix, 27–28
Middle East, 15, 158
Midland, Michigan, 90
Mifepristone. *See* contragestation
Miro, Carmen, xxv
Mishell, Daniel Jr., 92, 105
Misoprostol, 109, 110
Mississippi River, 176
Mitochondrial DNA, role in heredity, 38
Monarch butterfly, 155
Monder, Carl, 124
Morning-after pill. *See* emergency
contraception
Moscow, Russia, 23
Mozambique, 184, 185
Mumbai (Bombay), xx, 23
population growth, 194
urbanization, 20, 21
water problems, 157
Munich, Germany, 23
Murray, Tom, 42

Nairobi, Kenya, 23, 25, 184, 199
Nasser, Abdul Gamal, 158
National Academies of Sciences, 164
National Football League, 125
Nayar, Sushila, 81
NCAA, 125
Nehru, Jawaharlal, xiii
Nelson, Warren O., 74, 125
Nepal, 56, 111, 183
Netherlands, The, 7
New Delhi, xxv, 20, 23, 54, 79, 82
New paradigm, xvi, 204
New York Botanical Garden, 174
New York City, 20, 21, 151, 194, 201
Central Park, 179
research centers in, 44, 79, 88, 103, 121, 191,
Newfoundland, 171
Nigeria, 15, 99, 120
Nile perch, 178
Nile river, 158, 177, 182
Nobel Peace Prize, 148, 195
Nobel Prize in Physiology and Medicine, 200
Nogales, Arizona, 158
Nogales, Sonora, 158
Nordberg, Olivia Scheifflin, 179
Norgestrel, 93

Norgren, Tiana, 12
Norplant. *See* contraception
North Africa, 15, 53, 158
North America, 107, 166, 179
food subsidies, effect of, 156
global warming, effects of, 172
migration to, 22
total fertility rate, 15
North Atlantic herring. *See* Jacobsson, Jacob
North Atlantic Ocean, 172
North Atlantic Treaty Organization (NATO), 172
North Korea, 10,
Notestein, Frank, xxvii
Notre Dame University, 150
Nuclear energy, 166

Obstetrical toad, 57
Obstructed labor, 182
Official Development Assistance (ODA), 184
Ogino, Kyasaka, 69
Operation Crossroads, 171
Oppenheimer, W., 80
Organization of Petroleum Exporting Countries (OPEC), 166
Organon Company, 102, 105
Oral contraceptives. *See* contraception
Ortho-McNeil Company, 77, 85, 106, 140
Osteoporosis, 66, 135, 207
Ovarian cancer, risk reducing factors, 63
Ovulation, 35, 37, 45, 69
suppression of, 55, 99, 136
Oxford University, 195

Paddock, William and Paul, 145
Pakistan, 14, 26, 157
education project, 187
Paradise wydahs. *See* African weaver finches
Parathion, 197
Paredes, Mario, 122, 123
Paris, France, 23
Parke-Davis Company, 76, 108, 125
Parthenogenesis, 39–40, 71
Partition of British India, 23
Peking Union Medical School, 117
Perez Palacio, Gregory, 108, 109
Perfect Storm, The, 172
Pergonal. *See* fertility drugs
Periodic abstinence, 69